Play of Consciousness
(Chitshakti Vilas)

Swami Muktananda

**with an Introduction by
Gurumayi Chidvilasananda**

PUBLISHED BY SYDA FOUNDATION
SOUTH FALLSBURG, NEW YORK

A Note on the Translation

No translation can fully reproduce the flavor of a book in its original language. Swami Muktananda wrote Chitshakti Vilas *in a unique and highly personal style, which combines the poetic colloquialism of spoken Hindi with the technical language of the Indian scriptures. This new translation is an attempt to render Baba's writing as literally as possible into an English idiom. We have done our best to keep the flavor of the original while avoiding constructions which would sound strange to a non-Hindi speaking reader. The spirit which flows through this book is beyond language, and the experience of reading it has little to do with appreciation of its style. Still, we hope that this translation, besides being accurate, conveys some of the power and subtlety of Baba's original Hindi.*

(Swami) MUKTANANDA, (Swami) CHIDVILASANANDA, GURUMAYI, SHAKTIPAT, SIDDHA MEDITATION and SIDDHA YOGA are registered service marks of SYDA Foundation in the U.S.A. and may be registered in other countries.

Printed in the United States of America
Fifth Printing, 1990
No part of this book may be used or reproduced in any manner whatsoever without written permission except in the case of brief quotations embodied in critical articles and reviews. For information address SYDA Foundation, P.O. Box 600, South Fallsburg, New York 12779.

This book was previously published with a different translation: the abridged version published in 1971 under the title Guru *and the expanded version published in 1974 under the title* The Play of Consciousness.

LCCN: 78-62769
ISBN: 0-914602-37-3 (paperback)

About Swami Muktananda

Born in 1908 into a wealthy family in Mangalore, India, Swami Muktananda began his spiritual journey at the age of fifteen. A few years later he took the vows of a monk, and was given the name Muktananda.

For twenty-five years he traveled around India on foot, spending time with many of the renowned saints and meditation masters of his day. He mastered the classical systems of Indian philosophy, as well as Hatha Yoga and many other branches of spiritual and worldly science. In 1947 he met Bhagawan Nityananda, one of the great modern saints of India and a master of the Siddha tradition. After nine years of intense study under Nityananda's guidance, Muktananda reached the goal of spiritual practice—the state of Self-realization.

When Nityananda took *mahasamadhi* (died) in 1961, he passed on the power of the Siddha lineage to Muktananda. During the next twenty one years Swami Muktananda traveled widely, making several tours of the world. In those two decades, through his teachings and through the transmission of his spiritual energy, he initiated hundreds of thousands of people all over the world into meditation and the experience of their own innate perfection. Muktananda's students have established several hundred meditation centers around the world.

In May of 1982, five months before his death, Swami Muktananda installed Gurumayi Chidvilasananda as his successor, transferring to her all the power and knowledge he had received from his Guru. Gurumayi had known Baba since she was a young child; the last ten years of his life she worked with him daily, receiving his instructions and guidance.

Today Gurumayi continues Swami Muktananda's work, traveling widely in America, Europe, Australia, as well as her native India, bestowing her grace and spiritual energy to the thousands who come in contact with her.

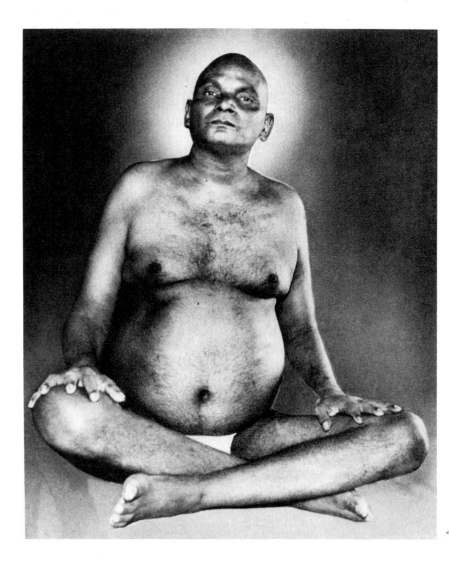

BHAGAWAN NITYANANDA

Foreword to the Second Edition
by Paul Zweig

Play of Consciousness is the spiritual autobiography of Swami Muktananda Paramahamsa, one of the great spiritual masters of our time. As such, it provides the answer to a question of extraordinary import to anyone concerned with the spiritual life: what sort of man is a Guru? What can he teach me, how did he learn what he knows? Swami Muktananda—Baba—answers by relating his own experience at crucial moments of his *sadhana* when, in flights of intense personal vision, he discovered that the scriptural texts of India, and of other religious traditions as well, provided a true anatomy of the inner life—a map of the spiritual journey such as only rare explorers have learned to know it.

Baba's account of his initiation by his Guru, Bhagawan Nityananda; of the visionary intensity which seized hold of him and progressively became focused into a palpable experience of God; of his harrowing temptations and the instruction he received from his Guru, has the feeling of an adventure story. But the story is not told for the sake of an exciting tale; nor, on the other hand, is it an explicit guide for the initiate to follow as he would follow a prescription. By describing the climax of his spiritual apprenticeship, Baba is giving us a glimpse of the inner country as he saw it; he is helping us to grasp the immensity of the task of *sadhana,* which each initiate performs according to his nature. He is letting us know that we live in a small portion of the mind, of the world, which we have grown so accustomed to that the merest step beyond it requires courage and guidance. In this sense, *Play of Consciousness,* in all its complexity and apparent strangeness, but also in its strong emotions, its honesty, is neither more nor less than a portrait of the God within.

Play of Consciousness is also an ecstatic hymn to Baba's Guru, Nityananda. It is, from beginning to end, the work of a disciple, and is therefore a moving lesson in the requirements of discipleship. Every page reminds us that devotion to the Guru is the key to all yogic discipline. It is the lever which *sadhana* applies to the fear-created habits of the mind. Love, which is another name for devotion, is the only cure for fear, and *sadhana,* as Baba describes it, is simply training in love, self-truth, spontaneity.

The inner unfolding of *sadhana* begins when the Guru, by the sheer touch of his personal being, triggers a flood of pent-up love, or spiritual energy—Kundalini—in his disciple. The Guru becomes the visible focus of that love, and he is, of all men, the complete, unwithholding lover. He becomes, for the disciple, a living reminder of the goal of *sadhana;* a visible example of what the disciple glimpses in himself now and then: that spontaneous, all-embracing Consciousness; that lucid unity of awareness, refusing nothing, accepting everything, which is the goal of Siddha Yoga.

By speaking as a disciple, Baba reveals the essential teaching—the "secret"—of Siddha Yoga, as he himself experienced it: that all the achievements of the spiritual path are contained in the disciple's love for his Guru. By identifying with his Guru, by opening his sensibility to his Guru's presence, by acting in accordance with his Guru's instructions, the disciple himself becomes the Guru. In Baba's definition, *sadhana* becomes an apprenticeship in self-knowledge, and, finally, in self-reliance, which means reliance on the underlying spontaneity, on the "inner Guru," which sustains all of mental life, and is the interior dimension of God.

Much of what Baba relates in *Play of Consciousness* has never been told by previous Masters to any but fully initiated disciples. He himself received only the most subtle, usually wordless guidance from his Guru. All that had generally been known of Siddha Yoga, and the phenomena of Kundalini awakening, had been provided by a few highly technical treatises which, however interesting from a philosophical point of view, were of little use in guiding the practical experience of individuals. In this sense, Baba made a radical departure from the traditional practice of Siddha Yoga. He did this at the bidding of his Guru, Bhagawan Nityananda, who told him that his work as a Siddha Master would be to teach the philosophy of Siddha Yoga to many people, and to guide their practical experience of *sadhana*.

Baba's task as a teacher brought him to the West three times. In a very few years, it turned Gurudev Siddha Peeth from a small three-room compound to a large international center where thousands of disciples pursue their *sadhana*. Siddha Yoga ashrams and meditation centers have been founded all over the world, so that disciples, while pursuing their lives at home, can also sustain and broaden their spiritual apprenticeship. *Play of Consciousness* has been translated into all the major European languages, and into many Indian languages as well.

One of Baba's important achievements as a teacher was to dissolve the exotic atmosphere usually attached to yoga and other Eastern disciplines. What he had to teach, he often said, was not Hinduism, but the Self; not to live in a cave wearing orange robes, but to see God in oneself as one is, and to see Him where one is, as a Christian, Jew or Moslem, as a business man, a parent, or a worker. That is why he chose to write directly and simply, avoiding the abstractions of philosophical discourse. As *Play of Consciousness* makes clear, a fully realized Master is one who has discovered in his own experience the origin of all philosophies. With him, traditions begin over again; and all the great spiritual texts are his own biography.

Contents

Book One: The Path of the Siddhas
Part 1: The Importance of God-Realization

Part 2: My Meditation Experiences

Book Two: Teachings of the Siddhas

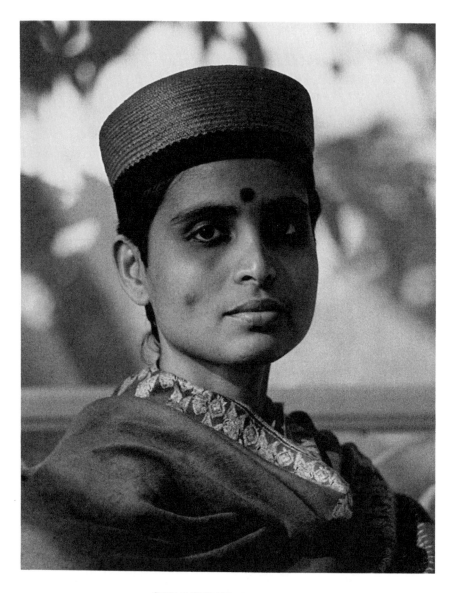

SWAMI CHIDVILASANANDA

Introduction

Play of Consciousness—what a beautiful name for a book. It is a description of that supreme state which Baba Muktananda attained and in which he lived throughout the remainder of his life.

The sages attempted to explain the supreme Truth in countless words which fill volumes. Nevertheless, they always kept the key to the direct experience of that Truth a secret between the Guru and the disciple. For this reason, even though you may read the scriptures again and again, you can never grasp from them the actual experience of the Truth. They repeat, "For that, you need a Guru." The extraordinary feature of *Play of Consciousness*, as many people have discovered, is that it can actually give the direct experience not only to one who reads it but often to one who merely glances at it or touches it.

Through the greatness of his heart and his compassion for humanity, Baba Muktananda has revealed in this book the highlights of his own spiritual *sadhana*. For this reason, you will find that its format differs from that of the ancient scriptures. Can spiritual experience be confined within a particular form? Nature always takes its own course: the wind blows, fire burns, and water flows—all in their own majestic ways. Similarly, everything that Baba has revealed to us in this book is an expression of the ever-changing dance of the universal Consciousness. Just as God has assumed countless forms in the outer universe, the inner experiences that He gives us are equally diverse. One of the *Shiva Sutras* says, *vismayo yogabhūmikāhā*—"The different stages of yoga are filled with wonders."

Every stage of a seeker's *sadhana* is an aspect of the supreme Truth. It isn't that every meditator has to have all the experiences that are so beautifully depicted in this book. Some meditators may not have any of them. But this does not mean that they are not making any progress. Spiritual experiences happen only for the benefit and growth of the seeker, and they vary according to the needs of each individual. As the awakened Kundalini purifies the seeker, it rids him of all his old impressions, blocks, and impurities. Because these differ from person to person, the process is unique for everyone. It is not necessary that everyone have dramatic physical *kriyas*. The Shakti is supremely intelligent and manifests in a way which is totally appropriate for each person. Just as the same food tastes different to all those who sample it, in the same way, this *prasad* which Baba Muktananda has offered us is experienced differently by each person who receives it.

Because *Play of Consciousness* is self-explanatory, I need not fill your mind with a detailed description of what it contains, nor will I attempt to analyze Baba's attainment point by point. What kind of meter do we have that could possibly do such a thing? In the words of Tukaram Maharaj, "For a person who has become a true friend of God, the creepers in his courtyard are like wish-fulfilling trees. As he strolls on his way, the stones in his path become wish-fulfilling jewels. The vastness of his knowledge cannot be denied. The *darshan* of such a being is truly rare. His casual conversation is more significant," says Tuka, "than the teachings of Vedanta."

Baba Muktananda was the embodiment of the supreme light. From his presence there constantly emanated rays of the power of meditation. His life has in turn given life to many. It has served as a torch illuminating our understanding of the glorious and awe-inspiring play of Consciousness.

SWAMI CHIDVILASANANDA

Dedication

My mother loved me very much, for I was her only son. She was a devotee of Lord Shiva, and it was her worship of Parashiva-Shakti which had given me to her, as a boon of His grace. But I could not give any happiness to my mother, nor could I make her contented. Instead, I left home when I was young and so caused her a lot of pain. She wasted away in grief for her lost son and finally died, remembering me all the time.

Children owe a great debt to their mothers. Mothers feed their children with their own vital juices; they give up their own happiness and find it in their children's happiness. What must my mother have done for her dear son! What ideas and plans she must have had for me! How many gods and goddesses she must have propitiated for the sake of my happiness! She must have asked all the astrologers, "What sort of wife will my son have? How many children will he have? Will he become famous? Will he go to other countries? How many factories will he open? Will his mother be a source of joy to him?" This is how a mother loves her children. If an astrologer says something ominous, she will immediately start propitiating all the gods; she will keep fasts not only on Thursdays, Fridays, and Saturdays, but every day if she can. When her child goes to school, she keeps thinking, "When is he coming home? Why hasn't he come yet?" She looks inside and outside, again and again. She looks at the clock. She waits for the sound of a car. "Why hasn't my child come?" A child is indebted to his mother for her infinite care of him. Still, the hard-hearted child leaves her, giving, in God knows how many ways, violent blows to her maternal affections.

My predicament was similar. I was slightly over fifteen when one day I left the love of my mother and father far behind. I should not have done such a thing. But what could I do? I was destined to behave so callously. It was supposed to happen, so it did. When I came to my senses, I remembered my mother. This was during the time of my *sadhana*, when I was a wandering *fakir* practicing the yoga of meditation and engaged in my studies on the spiritual path. How many mothers—from Yeola, Chalisgaon, Kasara, Kokamathan, Vajreshwari, and other places—have looked after me, giving me food and drink, clothes, things for my daily bath, and other necessities. They did everything for me in just the way that appealed to my temperament and suffered many hardships for it, for my nature was a bit fiery and I lacked patience. If they brought food at 11:15 instead of 11:00, I would fly into a rage, yelling, "Why are you late?" If it was brought five minutes early, I would get angry and shout, "Why are you so early?" During the period of my *sadhana*, my temperament was extremely peculiar and arrogant. Yet how much love these mothers gave me! They really are my revered mothers, who did so much for me. With hearts full of pure and selfless devotion they fed me and put up with my disposition. If the food was seasoned a bit too much or too little, I would not eat it. If it was too hot or too cold, I would want to know why. How shameful! Even I don't know why I was not able to bear even petty mistakes. I was merciless with them, I never excused them, and I felt no remorse about it. Those mothers served me with their own expense and toil, even neglecting their children for my sake, but still I had no compassion for them, no forgiveness. O Lord, why did you give me such an arrogant nature? I don't know.

All these mothers, including sweet, affectionate and loving mothers from Delhi and Bombay, still regard me as a temperamental child and give me their motherly affection with faith, devotion, and love. When I go on a journey, they come with me. Why? To cook Baba's food. When I go to Delhi, why do they come with me? To cook Baba's food. Even if I am traveling throughout the whole of India, I always eat at 11:30, so the mothers get up at 3:00 in the morning to prepare my food and put it in the car. I make it a strict rule to stick to the planned time of departure, so they have to get everything ready very quickly. Then the food has to be kept warm while we are on the road, so they use thermoses. Because tea has to be ready at 3:00 p.m., they take a stove and milk in the car with them so that while we are moving tea can be ready on time.

They have kept my filial affection alive by undergoing such hardships. Remaining unperturbed, they have borne my peculiar temperament and put up with my fastidious ways. This would not have been possible if a part of my real mother were not in them. Many mothers and their husbands have been good to me in many different ways. As I remember them, I beg them to forgive me generously. I bow to you, mothers, with all my heart, seeing you each as my own mother, the one who gave birth to me. I pray to Bhagavan Nityananda that I may always see in you that same mother, Goddess Chiti Kundalini, whom I love so much.

There is one mother here who has endured much hardship, taking care of me on my journeys as her own son. She was not strong, but she gave me great service. Her health was not good, but she was never lazy or negligent. She never thought of her own home. Her sons and daughters were studying in college, but she was not attached to them. She never worried about who would look after her home or what would happen to her life. She looked after Baba's food and his welfare for one, two, or even three months at a time in the blazing heat, the freezing cold, and the stormy monsoon. I dedicate this work to her, Shrimati Sharda Amma, who is as dear to me as a mother, in memory of my own holy mother, Kusumeshwari.

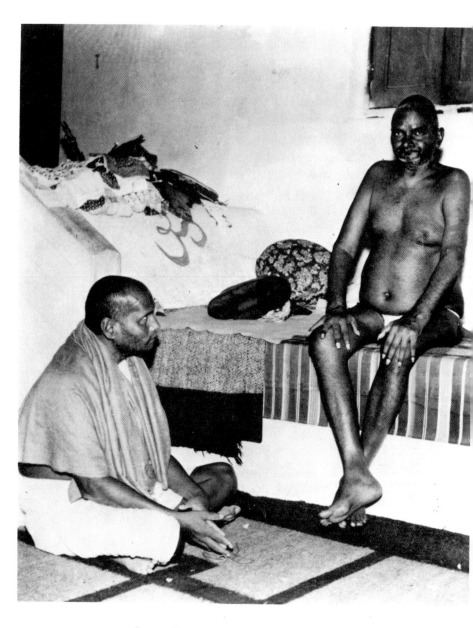

SWAMI MUKTANANDA AT THE FEET OF HIS GURU

Invocation

I invoke the lotus feet of Nityananda, the supreme Guru, who is the blessing of all blessings, whose glance destroys all misfortunes and bestows supreme good fortune.

I invoke the Guru, who is Parabrahman, the supreme Absolute, who is free from stain and completely pure, whose presence easily bestows the state of Parabrahman.

May Sri Nityananda, the goal of the meditations of the Siddhas, the foundation of Vedanta, the supreme Witness realized through the wisdom of detachment, give us his blessings.

May the supreme Guru, Sri Nityananda, by whose favor man acquires new awareness, who transmits his own inner Shakti into the disciple through Shaktipat and establishes him in a perfection like his own, award me full success in the composition of this work.

I bow to Sri Guru Nityananda, the lord of my heart, that he may give me his blessings—Nityananda, who lives in the world of Siddhas and yet pervades everywhere, who is the pure, conscious Self, the divine power of grace to his disciples, whose grace is itself the knowledge of the individual soul's identity with the Absolute.

I pray to Sri Guru Nityananda, that he may bring this work to completion—Nityananda, who lives in the hearts of Siddha students, who is their supreme beloved, who enters them and works within them through countless processes and movements.

For the perfection of my meditation, I bow to Sri Gurudev, the supreme father, who is beyond both diversity and unity, whose actions reveal equality and awareness of the Self of all, who easily bestows the state of perfection, and who is the guide of the Siddha Path.

O Sadguru, giver of grace! You yourself are the knowledge of perfection I received from you. You fully pervade everywhere, and Siddha students see you repeatedly in the Blue Pearl. O blue jewel, Bhagavan Sri Nityananda, I bow to your lotus feet.

You reveal yourself within the Blue Pearl the instant that the ignorant notion of "I and mine" is destroyed. Meditation on the Self is worship of you, repetition of the mantra *So'ham* is the invocation to you, and full surrender is the offering to you. The supreme bliss that pulsates in the wake of meditation is your pure essence. You are the adored deity of Siddha students, dwelling forever in the blue abode in the radiant cluster of Consciousness in the *sahasrara*.

May Sri Nityananda, the Self of all and the goal of "Thou art That," who dwells in Ganeshpuri and plays in the heart of Muktananda, shower on his Siddha students the nectar of supreme bliss and grant them eternal joy and everlasting peace.

Prayer to Sri Gurudev

This is my prayer to Sri Gurudev!

May everyone's life be a paradise.
May the trivial feeling of "I and mine" disappear,
And the knowledge of Chiti arise in our hearts.
May all beings always worship you with love and equanimity,
And the movement of our breath ever repeat the mantra So'ham.

Bless me, that I may worship you with the awareness of the Self of all.
May I abandon distinctions of race, religion, and language, and keep
*   my mind in purity.*
May I behold you, Gurunath, in the great and small, the suffering and
*   poor, the noble and foolish.*
Give me simplicity of mind, a humble spirit, and a generous heart.
May I be the bestower of true knowledge.

Grant me this boon, Gurudev:
May I always meditate on you in the temple of my heart.
O Self of all! May I always love the all-pervasive light.
May I be devoted to you, O Guru.
Let my awareness be steadfast in knowledge, yoga, and meditation.
May I ever be a worshiper of Siddha Vidya;
May my mind merge with Chitshakti.

May I always behold in you Rama, Krishna, Shiva, and Shakti.
May I live in Ganeshpuri, where your Siddha Yoga dwells.
Set me free from distinctions of country, language, sect, and race, and
*   give me equality of vision.*
Fill my heart with the pulsations of Nityananda.
May my mind be that of Nityananda.

May everyone attain simplicity, truth, courage, valor, discretion, and
*   radiance.*
May the world be a garden of joy for all, complete with the wishing
*   tree and the wishing cow.*
May Siddha students become masters of their senses and take delight
*   in Kriya Yoga.*
O Gurunath! May I always see you within the temple of the human
*   heart and feel fulfilled.*

Let me fulfill my duties so long as there is life in this body,
And let me remember you constantly.
Let my life be full of my own labor, Gurunath.
May I meditate on you always.
O Gurudev! Grant me this at least:
May I always be united with you.
May I behold you always and everywhere, from east to west, from
*   north to south.*

You are Parashiva, invisible and pure;
You are the very form of Satchidananda.
The universe is in you; you are in the universe;
There is no differentiation in you; you are unsurpassed, unique.
Muktananda says: Sri Gurunath! May the Siddha Science come to full
*   flower.*
May our meditation be dynamic.
May we find repose in the Blue Pearl.

May I always wander joyfully in the world,
And may you abide forever in my heart.
Muktananda says: O Gurunath! May our lives be the play of universal
*   Consciousness!*

Preface

I am a follower of the Siddha Path, and I am alive through the grace of a Siddha. My living, eating, bathing, meditation, mantra, breath, attainment, salvation, and repose are a Siddha's benediction. What more can I say?

Nityananda, who dwells in the world of Siddhas, the perfect lord of Siddha Yoga, the supreme Guru, is Muktananda's beloved deity and his innermost being. I live through the blessing of his grace. His gracious Shakti, the power of divine grace, has spread throughout my body and made its dwelling place within my heart.

No one living in the world should feel that the barren and joyless experiences of the world are for him and that yoga and meditation are for ascetics who have detached themselves from everything. It is quite possible for ordinary people to practice Siddha Yoga while carrying on their occupations. Today, there are many followers of the Siddha Science who live in the world; in former times, too, countless householders followed this path. They became ideal men and women, fully carrying out both their spiritual and worldly pursuits.

This path is open to everyone. There is an inner divine power within every man and woman, which the *Shiva Samhita* has described thus:

> *mūlādhārastha vahnyātmatejo madhye vyavasthitā*
> *jīvaśaktiḥ kuṇḍalākhyā prāṇākārātha tejasī*
> *mahākuṇḍalinī proktā parabrahmasvarūpiṇī*

sabdabrahmamayī devī ekānekāksharākrutiḥ
sakti kuṇḍalinī nāma visantantunibhā śubhā

It means that the Shakti, the great Goddess, is of the nature of Brahman, the Absolute. People call Her by the name of Kundalini. She resembles a lotus stalk and lies in the womb of the lotus of the *muladhara*. She is in a coiled form and is filled with golden radiance and luminosity. She is Parashiva's supremely fearless Shakti. It is She who lives in man and woman as the individual soul. She is of the form of *prana*. All letters from *"a"* to *"ksha"* arise from Her. I am describing Her in order that human beings may know this inner power and use Her while living in the world. Kundalini is the essence of *Om*. When She is awakened, lives which had seemed commonplace and arid, unenjoyable and frustrated, become gay and flourishing, filled with sweetness, contentment, and delight.

Kundalini is the Goddess Chiti, the joyous divine energy that unfolds the universe. She lives coiled up in the *muladhara* and keeps all the organs of our body functioning properly. When awakened by the grace of the Guru, She transforms the body and improves our daily lives according to our destinies. She generates a feeling of deep friendship among people, enables them to see the divine in one another, and thus turns the world into paradise. She makes perfect whatever is not perfect in our lives.

When this divine power enters a man in the form of grace, he is completely transformed. As he becomes fully aware of the pervasiveness of his own inner Shakti, he develops a deep love for his wife, and a selfless relationship with her. The knowledge arises within him that she is not a woman, but the divine Kundalini. As Chiti reveals Herself within a wife, complete faith in her husband and boundless love for him arise in her, along with the desire to serve. Through the influence of this power there dawns within her the perfect understanding that her husband is not just a man, but the embodiment of God. As the power of the Guru's grace penetrates a mother, her whole life is suffused with joy. As the Shakti saturates her, she gains knowledge of her children's true nature. She acquires the ability to perfect them in wisdom, courtesy, and the fullest expression of their talents. The moment the grace of the supreme Kundalini is bestowed on her in the form of Shaktipat, she is given the capacity to lead her children along the highest path. This knowledge is not imaginary nor is it something that is only said by Muktananda. A verse in the *Rudra-hridaya Upanishad* testifies to its truth: *rudro nara umā nārī tasmai tasyai namo namaḥ*—"Rudra is man, Uma is woman; praise to him, praise to her."

The understanding arises that the primordial, eternal Truth—God, the Witness of all, the fundamental cause of the universe, the noblest object of worship, attributeless, formless, unborn, and without beginning—manifests as man, the husband, while Kundalini—God's supreme Shakti, who animates the world and who is called Chiti, Uma, Durga, Pratibha, Malti—appears as woman, the wife. I offer my salutations to both of them. Kundalini is the beloved queen of Parashiva and is half of his body. She becomes Radha, Sita, Mira, and takes the roles of daughter, housewife, mother, yogini, genetrix. Thus, people have a new awareness. When you obtain the Shakti of the Guru's grace, the world becomes heaven. This book has been written to demonstrate this.

May this supreme Shakti spread throughout all humanity. May all people flourish in the expansion of Chiti's play. May man and woman assimilate this Shakti and love each other completely, not with self-interested love, but with perfect knowledge. May they attain the play of Chiti, which is unfolded within, and become the embodiment of light. May wife and husband see each other, not as playgrounds of sensuality, but as worthy of each other's respect and reverence. May all the women of the world see the Shakti growing within, perceive the great glory of the Shakti, and understand their husbands as perfect rays of the same supreme Shakti. May they realize that true religion is the spirit of reverence, friendship, and devoted service, and thus become devout. This is the hope of Muktananda.

Every man and woman who lives in the world should remember another thing: the entire phenomenal universe is pervaded by Goddess Chiti. Chiti is the originator and sustainer of the world; the world exists within Her being.

Chiti is Paramashiva Paramatman—that which transcends the universe, which is perfect being, without attributes, the foundation of all things, the goal of the *neti neti*—"not this, not this," spoken of in

Vedanta, the basis of the knowledge *aham brahmasmi*—"I am the Absolute," the conscious Self. The supreme Shakti is inseparable from Paramashiva, who is absorbed in Her. She is also called Shiva-Shakti. It is Her beauty that is revealed in this phenomenal universe, animate and inanimate. She is the power of consciousness of the supreme Being and is completely identical with Him. The perceivable universe is the outer expansion of Her own inner pulsation.

She reveals Herself in every visible activity in life. She appears in various forms, favorable or unfavorable, helpful or obstructive. The *Pratyabhijnahridayam* says: *tannānā anurūpagrāhyagrāhakab-hedāt*—"She becomes manifold in the variety of mutually related objects and subjects." Revealing Herself in this way, supremely free Chiti becomes the thirty-six principles of creation through Her own will. She appears as masculine and feminine, or Purusha and Prakriti. Of the many differentiations in the world, these are the main two—Purusha and Prakriti, masculine and feminine. These distinctions pervade everything. Birds, animals, and trees are also divided into these two categories. In other activities, too, there is a dual distinction which permeates infinite forms: high and low, virtue and sin, bondage and liberation, ecstasy and anxiety, and so on. Yet it is the same Chiti that has become the perceiver and the perceived. What I wish to convey is that the world is permeated by Chiti, belongs to Chiti, *is* Chiti. If you see with the eyes of true knowledge, you will find nothing but Chiti in the world.

A person may or may not understand this. But even if his inner Shakti is not awakened, he should remember one thing: God dwells in the world in human form. According to the *Pratyabhijnahridayam: manusyadehamāsthāya chhannāste paramesvarāh*—"God takes on a human body and conceals Himself within it." Since it is God who dwells in the body, it follows that an aspirant of Siddha Yoga can easily unfold his inner Shakti.

When this is the case, how mistaken are people of the world who lack the knowledge of Chiti, who do not perceive Her, who do not adore Her within themselves. Even though the pervasion of Shiva-Shakti may seem to an ordinary person to be duality, to one who depends on the Guru's grace, it appears only as the perfect embodiment of love and non-duality. O voyagers in the world! If you want your journey to be free of obstacles, become aware of your venerable Goddess, Chiti Kundalini. Awaken Her with meditation, behold Her everywhere, and live in happiness. The forms of Gurus are Her blissful luster. I define this great Shakti Kundalini, who is the embodiment of Parabrahman, as Chitshakti. Chiti Kundalini, awakened through your Guru's blessing, will bring your journey smoothly to its completion. The great yoga of meditation will guide you on the spiritual path. With Chiti's blessing, you will become great. Your life will be filled with yoga, with delight and strength, with that which is beneficial as well as that which is pleasant. Your house will become Kashi, a place of pilgrimage, your work a daily ritual, your friends gods and goddesses, your meals sacred offerings. Everything that you do will become worship of the supreme Self. In due course of time, you will attain the final fruit—you will become merged in Chiti.

O Goddess Chitshakti! O Mother! O Father! You are Shakti. You are Shiva. You are the soul vibrating in the heart. Your manifestations—as the world and as the Self—are both filled with bliss and beauty. As long as they lack full knowledge of You, ignorant people project onto You various dualistic ideas such as Shiva-Shakti, world-illusion, bondage-liberation, indulgence-renunciation, spiritual-worldly. O supremely worshipful Mahashakti! When You take the form of the Guru to bless the disciple and enter within him, he realizes through inner knowledge that the external world is also Your play. Siddha Yoga, Kundalini, sublime worship, and the yoga of meditation are all created by You, and You permeate them all completely. They are the means through which You bring the *sadhana* of meditation to its fulfillment and grant the state of Your own nature.

Just as threads are present throughout a piece of cloth, just as clay is still clay when it is made into a pot, so this whole animate and inanimate universe is You Yourself. When one realizes this, one sees unity in the midst of differences and God in the midst of daily life. O Parashakti of Parashiva! When aspirants remember You while reciting *Namah Shivaya, So'ham,* or *Om,* and completely forget themselves, You reveal Yourself within them. O free, supreme Creator! All mantras are Your names and all rituals Your actions. The world is Your visible form. O universal Consciousness! This universe, which is full of different forms, different colors, different shapes, and an endless combination of different objects, is Your outward pulsation. I bow to You again and again.

A ray is no different from the sun, a wave is no different from the sea, bits of earth are no different from the earth, and You, Goddess Chiti, manifest Yourself in a multitude of forms. One ray from Your sheaf of rays, no different from You, is Your Muktananda. Muktananda arose from You, he lives in You, and in the end he will be absorbed in You. He is Your freedom, freed by You, and free in You. This book, presented with countless prostrations, is my offering to You.

My dear students of Siddha Yoga lovingly requested me to write about my own experiences during my *sadhana*. Subsequently, because of the persistence of my dear Amma, I began to write this book on Monday, May 12, 1969, at Shri Anandabhavana in Mahableshwar.

The subject and nature of this little book are not the same as the works of great beings of ancient times. Those books have their own great importance. Everything in this book is the work of Chiti. It is Chiti's gift and Chiti's creation. Siddha Yoga belongs to Goddess Chiti. The aim of this book is attainment of Chiti, and the name *Chitshakti Vilas* automatically sprang forth; it was not thought out.

Part 1
The Importance of God-Realization

God is all-pervasive, perfect, and eternal. He is in all things, both within
and without. He is immanent in all beings and lives in the temple of
the heart in the form of the inner Self. Yet there are few who know
Him. Many deluded people do not believe that He exists—in the heart
or anywhere else on this earth—for nowadays faith in God is regarded
as false. Certain materialistic philosophies hold that the origin of
creation is in nature, that the universe has no creator and is just an
aggregation of atoms and molecules. Some people believe that God
lives in some far-off Vaikuntha or Kailasa, or in the fifth or the seventh
heaven, and that He is not manifest in the heart. There are also modern
thinkers who question the existence of God because of the conflict,
suffering, and misery they see in the world. In one place there are
floods, in another drought; in one place famine, in another surplus.
"Why," they ask, "do we see so much inequality? The rains do not
come in time. There is no water to drink—only the tears that flow
from the eyes. There is not enough grain for food—nothing to eat but
the leaves of plants and trees. There are no houses to live in, there are
no clothes to cover one's nakedness. Why is there such adversity?"
Harboring such ever-increasing doubts, the hearts of these people
become dry and faithless.

Yet there are many countries in the world that have plenty of
food, wealth, and prosperity. The reason for this is their unrelenting
application, their constant industry. Japan is a small country without

much fertile soil, yet it is self-sufficient in food because its people have completely and with total faith dedicated themselves to the art of agriculture. An Indian proverb says, "The python does no service, the bird does no work," but people like the Japanese do not believe in such indolence. If people live lives devoid of responsibility and full of laziness, and then turn against God saying, "If God exists, why are we hungry?"—isn't that just a mockery? Belief in God should not be used for your own self-interest, which means that you should not make a business of it in order to make your life complete. God exists, but man is in a sad state because he has turned away from Him and lives without faith.

I once met a family in which there were seven doctors, each a specialist in a certain field. A boy in this family fell ill because he ate the wrong things. He took the medicine prescribed for him but he did not change his diet. He got worse and was put in the care of another doctor. Is it right to doubt that the medicine of the doctors in his family was effective? The truth is that man gets the fruit of his actions from God, and the fruits correspond to the nature of his actions.

If you want to know God, theories and speculations are of no use. He is perfectly manifest, but in a subtle form. He is the unmoving foundation of all our actions, inward and outward. There are many marvelous places in India, many abodes of Siddhas. Can we see all of them? We cannot, but this does not mean that such places do not exist. In the same way, a great and divine Shakti is manifest within us, working ceaselessly. To say that it does not exist is naive rationalism. It is God, the creator, who has made this world a good place to live in, by forming the outer world and the inner world in His own image, and then pervading both. If God were not in the world, who could live there? Who would strive to make his worldly dealings honest and pure? If the world is interesting and full of joy, it is because of God. His glory is boundless, and it is because of the existence of the infinite One that we experience His taste and His sweetness. It is only because the bliss of the supremely blissful Lord is reflected in the world that we derive a little satisfaction from all sense pleasures and from all worldly actions. We find the shadow of God's bliss in the taste of food, in the sweetness of water, in the melodies of the *ragas* and *raginis,* in the soft smile of blossoming flowers, and in the squeals of small children. If God's radiance were not in the beauty of many-colored flowers, why should we be so captivated by them, why should we love them so? If mangoes, pineapples, tangerines, or pomegranates lacked His beauty, sweetness, and savor, why should they taste so sweet to us? Their sweetness and nectarean savor are due to that divine principle. There is so much sweetness in plain and pure water! How we love the sun, its bright rays of many colors! At the touch of these delicate rays, lotuses open, plants sway with happiness, the whole kingdom of birds is filled with bliss and begins to sing. Look carefully, look with subtlety: these sunrays, these creepers, surrender to each other in mutual love and sacrificial worship, and meet each other with silent speech. What divine music there is in the gently flowing wind; what a sweet, cool, happy touch! All this is the love-flow of God manifest. But because man is deprived of the recognition of God, he sees the universe, which is the embodiment of Consciousness, as something quite different. In his ignorance, he perceives only defects.

This world is a perfect reflection of God. The Vedantic teaching: *sarvam khalvidam brahma*—"All this is indeed the Absolute"—is the ultimate truth. Everything is God. All countries, all holy places, all names are God's. Only in the eyes of men are there differences of high and low. Truly, all the regions of this earth are holy places of the Lord. All bodies of water are holy rivers of God. All the shapes and forms of the world contain the very sound of God's name. Endless is the glory, endless are the names, endless is the sport of the Infinite. There is no end to God. However much you read, there is something left to study. However many holy places you visit, there are still more left to see. However far you see, there is always more ahead. Such is the pervasiveness of the divine principle, the divine vastness; more divine than the divine is His glory.

Our lives are so short, our bodies so ephemeral, and this world so full of hazard and suffering that it is absolutely necessary to find God. But the way to Him is very hard. Just as man has a bloodline, so the divine principle has a lineage. This world descends from God, who is without beginning. To doubt and speculate about this is not right. One seed produces another identical seed. The ones yet to come will have the same nature as the first. In this way, Brahman is gradually born from Brahman. The Self of every man is an integral portion of

One

The Necessity of Meditation for Happiness in the World

There are so many things inside the human body. If, even once, man could discover his body in meditation, truly he would benefit a great deal from it. Who knows what there is in this body! There are so many *chakras* just in the head, so many different springs welling with nectar, so many clusters of nerve filaments, so many kinds of musical harmonies, so many different fragrances; there are rays from so many different suns, abodes of so many different deities. Though all this is inside him, man, tragically caught in his delusion, indulges himself in the arid world outside. It has become a common practice of man's life to behave like a dog who gnaws away on the dry shell of a bone, but does not gain anything from it. On the contrary, it drinks only the blood that runs from its own jaws. Like a dog, man digs for joy in the external world, but what does he get in the end? Only toil and dryness.

The inner world is far greater than the outer world. How extraordinary is the place of clairaudience in the ear, how significant the center of sleep in the throat! It is here that the fatigue of the waking hours is dissolved, for no matter what man acquires in the waking state, at the end of the day all that he has attained is weariness. Man can ride on a horse or an elephant or recline on a palanquin or any other vehicle, but at the end of the day he is tired. He may acquire wealth, gold, and a kingdom, but at the end of the day he has found only lassitude. He can see dramas, all the beauty of the world, vaults of rubies and pearls, but at the end of the day he is weary. He can win all titles, all honors, but at the end of the waking state it is Shramaraj, the lord of tiredness, who welcomes him. Even if he becomes the lord or ruler of the universe, he will still get tired.

When you go to sleep to remove your fatigue, at night or during the day, it is in the throat center that your fatigue is dispelled. Only there do you fall asleep. My dear ones! Before you go to sleep, you take off all your ornaments, because nothing that you have earned is of any use to you while you sleep. If you even remember your cherished possessions or wealth, your sleep is interrupted. Sleep comes only when you forget your riches; if you cannot forget, then you take refuge in a sleeping pill. When you get up, you feel happy and dynamic. If you cannot sleep, you become restless, maddened, and tormented. This proves that sleep is a treasure, which lives in the throat center and which I call Shveteshwari, the white goddess. Here is located the *vishuddha chakra,* with its presiding deity. If you do not see this throat center, where supremely joyous sleep is found, what will you understand of your own body?

In the heart center there is a lotus. Each petal of this lotus has its own quality: desire, anger, infatuation, greed, love, modesty, knowledge, detachment, joy, omniscience, etc. Within the heart is a space the size of a thumb, and here a divine light shimmers. The sages have spent their lives looking at this light. How marvelous is the heart center! How magnificent is the light in the heart space! How divine is the Goddess Kundalini! As She unfolds, man's entire being is transformed.

O man, when you have this infinite storehouse of qualities within you, what kind of happiness are you looking for in the external world? You do not meditate, you do not perform good actions, you do not take care of your precious body—how can you find happiness without doing these things?

O unconscious man, wake up, meditate; not just for liberation, not just out of religious duty, not just for the laurels of yoga, not just to become praiseworthy, but at least, meditate to satisfy your desire for worldly objects.

You have been searching for beauty in all four directions but you have not found it, and you have become tired. You look for happiness in movies and theater, you wander for it from country to country, and still you do not find it. What happens in the end? Looking for beauty you lose your own beauty and become ugly; looking for happiness you find hardship and weariness. Now tell me—how much sincerity is there in your search?

Tell me more. You search for savor in various foods—in tea, coffee, Coca-cola, puddings. You go to restaurants and nightclubs. What do you actually get? In the search for joy, you yourself become joyless. Your face shrivels, your money gets spent. In place of joy you get disease. Your life passes by. Cooking and tasting all kinds of delicacies, you destroy your own sense of taste. Even the sweetness that was already there disappears. You do not find the real, joyful, pure, and precious nectar that is in your heart.

The same thing happens in quest of smell. You look for enjoyment in the latest perfumes, in sweet-smelling flowers; you apply the choicest scents from Paris. While you pursue fragrance you become old, and eventually you find only stench. O man, meditate a little and see. You will find that at the place where the nose meets the eyebrows there is incomparable fragrance. Brother, in this place even bad smells are transmuted into pleasing aromas. There, the individual soul becomes full of the greatest bliss.

Then you search relentlessly for delight in sound, in words. You hope that everyone will address you with courteous words. Who knows how many people you have tried to please, how many you have enticed for the sake of words? You look in the newspaper to see what has been written about you, how much praise you have received. You spend money and secretly commission a book to be written about yourself, and when nobody buys it, you give it away free. How mad you are to hear praise! "What did my wife say? What did they say about me in that meeting?" Yet, though nice words please you, you do not find true happiness in them. Your body is not vigorous. Rays of light do not shine from your face. You listen to good music, you learn *ragas* and *raginis,* but the bud of love inside you still does not bloom. You do not hear that word which the saints have heard and spoken of: *so'ham śabdāchi ṭhāīṁ pahuḍat jhāloṁ*—"I found rest in the word *So'ham*," and in the end you lose it. O soul of man, where are you going? You have heard everything, but you have not heard the word from the Guru's mouth. You have not heard the word by which you can drink the elixir of immortality, by whose potency the light of a new awareness begins to shine throughout your world.

And look what you do to satisfy the sense of touch: you go completely mad. You try soft cushions, clothes, beds strewn with flowers, but you don't find satisfaction. You look for it in velvet clothes, but you don't find it. You look for it even where it doesn't exist. Engaged in this search, you find another human form just like yours, and in it you seek the pleasure of touch, but you don't find it there either. Even that touch does not bring you comfort. You devote your life to the pursuit of touch, but you find nothing, and in the end your sense of touch becomes dulled. O unfortunate one, if your inner Shakti were awakened, the touch of the ever-blissful Parashakti would spread throughout your body. You would become an ocean of the joy of touch.

Muktananda says: O people, meditate, even to find the prized objects of your senses that you are looking for in the world, for these pleasures are all inside you, and you will find them there. Your world will then become full of delight; your life will become heavenly. When through God's grace this inner Shakti is awakened, meditation begins to happen. Love the Shakti and honor your Self. Meditate within. Meditate on the inner Shakti by whose power you consider yourself "you." Meditate on Her by whose grace you love each other and surrender your souls to one another as husband and wife. The gracious and divine Shakti lives in both of you as your very own form. She is the same Shakti that Muktananda adores.

It doesn't matter which sect you belong to, for none has forbidden meditation on the Self; therefore, meditate. O men and women, no matter which caste you belong to, meditate on the supreme inner Shakti. No matter which country you belong to, meditate on the Shakti of the Self. O simple-hearted people, no matter which political party you belong to, the practice of meditation will not be an obstacle. Do not consider a sect, party, country, religion, or degree a hindrance to inner meditation. Do not consider the position of a leader, official, swami, or head of a monastery as an obstacle. Meditate. Even if you're a *mandaleshwar*, meditate. Don't consider your position to be an impediment to meditation. If it is, what is the use of your petty position? Whether you are a boy or a girl, a man or a woman, a celibate, a householder, a recluse, or a *sannyasi*—meditate. Seek your own Self; you will find it. Meditate on your own Self—in your house if you live in a house, in the forest if you live in a forest, in the city if you live in a city, in the village if you live in a village, or wherever you may live. Meditate, all of you, whether you are a patient or a doctor, whether you are a defendant or a lawyer, whether you are a beggar or a rich merchant. Whether you have good qualities or bad, whether you are virtuous or sinful—meditate. You will find the peace of your Self. The culmination of your search for the objects of the five senses lies in meditation. The culmination of your pursuit of art, poetry, dance, and liberation also lies in meditation.

As you continue to meditate, the Shakti will soon open Her hidden storehouses, and then you will immediately get higher meditation. When that happens, your true beauty will be revealed. You will come to know those divine lights that exist inside you. Because of their existence your fleshly body becomes beautiful, because of their captivation you feel mutual love for one another. With the appearance of dazzling divine light during meditation, your first worldly desire—beauty—will be fulfilled; your treasured beauty will be attained. Compared to that inner light even the beauty of the god of love is minimal, and it is this light that husband and wife will see shining in each other. When this beauty is revealed to you, you will find your precious object; you will see the whole world as full of brilliance.

When beauty is revealed, its companion, sound, arises. As sound emanates, you hear sweet and divine music. The treasure of *nada,* which is filled with infinite virtues, will arise in your head. You will get deep and pleasant sleep, such as even the gods enjoy. Listening to this music, you will dance. It will chase away your indifference, your apathy, the worries of your mind, and the disease of erratic thinking. It will make the world look fresh and green. O voyagers of the world! The music on the radio, the news of different places, and conversation will all seem bland. You will save yourself the expense of radio and television.

Not only this, but the sound will make you taste a divine elixir. The elixir released by this sound drops from the palate and is very beautiful. It is sweeter than the sweetest. Each drop is worth millions.

It is worthy of being treasured by everyone. By taking it you get rid of all sickness. As you taste it, you will be filled with joy, and afterward you will find that taste in whatever you eat or drink, whether it is cooked or uncooked, simple or dry. There will be no more suffering, no more want, no more feeling of "I and mine." You yourself will become the vessel of this elixir, and subsequently you will find the elixir of love in your husband, your wife, and your children. *Raso vai saḥ rasaṁ hyevāyaṁ labdhvānandī bhavati*—"Indeed, He is the elixir by obtaining which, one experiences bliss within." This is the essence of the gods, the essence of love, the essence of yoga, and the essence you have been searching for in the world. Without it your life is as joyless, parched, and barren as chaff. Look, the world that is now without joy will become full of delight, and along with that your own life will also become full of happiness.

O brothers! There is also fragrance. Where there is beauty, sound, and taste, there is always the fourth brother, fragrance. When the divine scent that is inside man reveals itself, the entire world becomes perfumed, and the same fragrance spreads throughout your house. As you sense this divine aroma in others, your mind becomes peaceful. Heaviness and dullness leave your body, and every limb is supercharged with vitality. Then even if you lack things in life, you will feel fullness everywhere. You will feel divine love pulsing inside for your children and relations and teachers. You will sing that the world itself is full of love and equanimity.

O man! There is the fifth object of your search, touch. You go through a lot for its sake. You crave pleasure, peace, and bliss through touch. You seek it in your beautifully adorned wife, but find only feverish heat. You touch her for perfect bliss, but get only perfect agitation. You don't attain bliss at all. However, when your inner Kundalini Shakti unfolds, Her love will flow all through your body, through all the 72,000 *nadis*. Her rapture will spread through every particle of blood, as a result of which you will experience bliss in every pore. Then your desire for the joy of touch will be satisfied and your world filled with sweetness, bliss, and love. Consequently, the light that was lost will return to your eyes, your lips will become red, your dried-up face will become aglow with love, and will blossom. You will experience happiness in everything. Wives will become goddesses to their husbands, husbands gods to their wives. Sons will become gods, daughters goddesses. Mothers-in-law will become goddesses, fathers-in-law gods, and neighbors as well will become divine. Houses will become temples. God will not only be in the temple; you yourself will become God. You will behold exquisite beauty, you will taste nectar, smell fragrance, hear divine sound, and find joy in touch. In this way, how happy your life will become! You will sing:

Avaghāchi saṁsāra sukhāchā karīna
ānandeṁ bharīna tinhī loka

(Saint Jnaneshwar)

We will make the whole world full of happiness.
We will show that all the three worlds are full of bliss and nothing but bliss.

God is in the forest, God is in the mind, God is in ourselves, we ourselves are in God. We belong to God alone. Saying this you will dance all day in the love of God. You will repeat as a mantra, "God is the husband, God is the wife, God is the intellect, God is the goal." You will understand that God is on all sides, the whole world belongs to God, and God maintains it. Dear people of the world! Thus your house will become a place of pilgrimage and both husband and wife will become divine. Your household chores will be an act of worship, and your worldly life will become your duty to God.

Muktananda says: Meditate for this purpose. Your daily needs are fulfilled in meditation, and meditation is also the place of rest from everyday life. Meditation is your friend, your guide, your wishful-filling cow, and your wish-fulfilling tree. Therefore, practice meditation a little every day.

Two

Spirituality in Worldly Life

If man combined his worldly life with meditation and did his *sadhana* of meditation at the same time as his daily commitments, then the world, which had been filled with the threefold agony—the physical and mental suffering caused by oneself, by others, or by fate and the forces of nature—would become heavenly. It is simply because man is indifferent to God that the world is full of pain and suffering for him. If you made a sweet pudding, full of delicious ingredients—pistachios, almonds, cardamon—but left out the sugar, how could it have any taste? In the same way, the world can be enjoyable only if you meditate on God. Through meditation man can make the world his greatest friend; without meditation on God, the world is full of suffering and pain. The truth is that life in the world can be a magnificent way to happiness, but only if God is in it completely. Without remembrance of God, without knowledge of Him, without meditation on Him, worldly life is crippled; it has no savor, no delight.

Don't abandon the world and your near and dear ones. Don't waste your strength running in every direction in search of God. Don't lose yourself while you look for peace and rest. Beloved people, stay at home with your husbands, your wives, your children. Be friendly with your crafts, skills, and talents. Stay with your businesses and factories. According to destiny, you may be a rich man or a laborer, a king or a beggar, but God belongs to everyone. God belongs to the poor as much as to the rich, to housewives as much as to the *gopis* of

Vraja, to ordinary people as much as to the ancient saints, sages, yogis, and yoginis. Call on Him with love, meditate on Him with love, and He will reveal Himself within you. You will see the divine light filled with His love. Cool streams of peace and the nectar of love will begin to flow in you from the *sahasrara,* and you will feel that you yourself are the incarnation of ecstasy. Not only this, but your body will become transformed. Then you will feel, "Indeed, I am that Shiva, I am that Rama, I am that Shyama. I am." You will start singing this song with love. Your former weeping and wailing of many lifetimes will be destroyed. Your lamentation, "I am unhappy, I am a sinner, I am poor," will end.

Don't consider your body to be just a mound of flesh formed of the seven elements. When it is not solely a place for the gratification of the senses, it is something wonderful. All holy places, all gods, all mantras, and all sites that bestow extraordinary powers are in it. I heard an old but true story from Bhagavan Nityananda. A couple once vowed to bathe in all holy places, to go around the whole earth, and to worship all the gods, but for some reason they could not carry out this vow. They worried and worried about this, until eventually they went to see a noble saint of great learning and experience and told him about their vow. The wise man said, "Don't worry. Not far from here is a couple who have become fully united with God and whose lives in this world are filled with Him. Through meditation they have awakened their inner Shakti, they have completely purified the centers of all the mantras and deities in the six *chakras,* and through their dedicated practice of the great yoga, Kundalini yoga, they have become God. They are holy people. Mahashakti Chiti plays within them. They appear to be ordinary human beings, but Chiti pervades their blood and all the fluids of their bodies. All sacred places and all deities are found in them. They are completely absorbed in the supreme Lord. Go there, walk around them three times, make them an offering, and think of them with your hearts full of love; then your vow will be fulfilled."

That is perfectly true. O dear man! God lives within you, as do all holy places, all mantras, all seed syllables, all deities. He is as much within you as He is in Kailasa or Vaikuntha. Why exhaust yourself looking for Him in different lands rather than within yourself? Lead your normal life and follow your own religions, but always place God first. Do not allow the teachings of any sect or devotional system to force you into thinking of yourself as ordinary, trivial, stupid, or weak. Do not lead yourself into destruction, don't bring about your own downfall, by saying that the body is without God. Don't make yourself an assassin of the soul by thinking that you are just ordinary. Don't kill yourself with your own hand by making yourself out to be insignificant and ignorant. Remember this saying of the Lord: *ātmaiva hyātmano bandhurātmaiva ripurātmanaḥ (Gita, 5:3)—* "You yourself are your own friend and your own enemy." Knowing this, quickly begin the search for your spiritual welfare. To make your way in the world you have searched out different colleges, you have searched in England and America, and at the end of your search you have acquired knowledge and become an engineer, a lawyer, a doctor, or a professor. Similarly, to find the peace of the Self, to make your house into a temple of yoga, and to attain Shiva even while being a lawyer, a doctor, or an engineer, you must go and search for a Guru.

Three

The Greatness of the Guru

Realization of God is possible only through a Guru. Illuminated with knowledge, the Guru is a descendant of Parabrahma. We should acquire the sublime grace of such a Guru, for until the Kundalini Shakti is awakened by the Guru's grace, our inner light does not shine, the inner eye of divine knowledge does not open, and our state of bondage cannot be lifted. In this limited condition, it is not possible to enjoy the divine experience of Godhood, for just as in a dream a king becomes a beggar and believes "I am a beggar," so in the sleep of ignorance the Self becomes limited and in that impoverished state believes that it is itself the doer and the experiencer, believes itself to be small and insignificant, and thus continually experiences suffering. Therefore, to develop inwardly, to attain divinity, and to arrive at the state of Parashiva, a guide is absolutely necessary—a Sadguru who knows the truth perfectly, who has spiritual power. Just as there can be no life without *prana,* so without the Guru there can be no knowledge, no unfolding and growth of the Shakti, no destruction of darkness, no opening of the third eye. The Guru is more necessary than a friend, a son, a husband, or a wife; more necessary than wealth, machines, factories, art, or music. What more can I say? The Guru is more necessary than health and *prana* itself. By his grace alone, the inner Shakti is unfolded. The glory of the Guru is full of mystery and is supremely divine. He gives a new birth to man, he gives him the experience of knowledge, he shows him *sadhana* and makes him a lover of God.

There are many gurus in the world. Everyone becomes a guru.
Wherever you go there are nothing but gurus—so many that people
have become fed up with all their conflicting teachings. Whenever a
guru appears, he starts up a new sect. He has never been anybody's
disciple but he claims to be everybody's guru. There are countless
teachings, countless sects. It has become a way of earning a living, a
business that doesn't involve any hard work. But this is not how it
should be.

A true Guru awakens the inner Shakti of a disciple and makes him
revel in the bliss of the Self. This is what the Guru really is: he is the
one who awakens the inner Shakti Kundalini through Shaktipat, who
sets the divine Shakti in motion in man's body, who gives instruction
in yoga, who bestows the ecstasy of knowledge and the joy of divine
love, who teaches detachment in action and grants liberation in this
very lifetime. That supreme Guru is identical with Shiva. That Guru is
Shiva, that Guru is Rama, that Guru is Shakti, that Guru is Ganapati,
that Guru is your father and mother. He is a descendant in the line of
Guruhood that began with Shiva, the primordial Guru. He is worthy
of being worshipped by all. He makes the light blaze in the body of his
disciple, gives him his blessing and grace, and then remains immersed
in his own sport. Through the favor of the Guru, man takes on the
form of God and lives drunk with ecstasy. Such a Guru is great and
exalted; he cannot be understood by the ordinary intellect.

The Guru understands the ways of the world very well. He knows
fully the laws of destiny. He possesses complete knowledge of God.
Adept in spiritual matters, he is just as clever in practical affairs. Disciples who live under the protection of such a Guru pass through the
most acute difficulties with ease, and seekers in a Siddha ashram live
fearlessly even in the most terrifying circumstances.

The devotees of our worshipful Guru Nityananda were fearless
because of him. Bhagavan Nityananda was a supremely divine Guru.
He lived in great secrecy, and his glory was not of an ordinary kind.
He would grant the experience of paradise to his devotees in their
own homes. Through his grace alone, without any strenuous disciplines, this great being would transform his devotees into yogis,
and seekers into priests of love. By his grace, he made his devotees

perceive knowledge and showed them God in the world. His teaching to men and women was: *paraspara devo bhava*—"Look upon each other as God." He was a perfect Siddha, one of the greatest Siddhas of Siddhaloka. The qualities of knowledge, yoga, devotion, and selfless action were perfectly blended in him. Though a yogi of great skill, he lived in a simple and ordinary way. He always lived in a thought-free state, as if his mind itself had become pure Consciousness. People knew Nityananda as a unique, ecstatic yogi. Although omniscient, he feigned ignorance. Everyone called him "Baba."

He did not attach any importance to *siddhis,* miraculous powers; he believed that compared with God's miracle of self-manifestation, all other miracles are insignificant. The world is in God. What miracle could be greater than this? Yet, sublime, wondrous, and secret powers lived in him, for it is quite natural for *siddhis* to live in Siddhas. They become active in such beings without being invoked and keep dancing around them unbidden. Even the earth considers herself fortunate when such perfect saints walk on her.

Bhagavan Nityananda was an extraordinary being and was renowned in the world. People will remember him, tell stories of his virtues, and see him in visions as long as the sun and moon shine. He was a glorious being who was worthy of the greatest honor, for he was the perfect embodiment of Guruhood. Singing his praises and remembering him, receptive people would get Shaktipat. Even now, Shakti is received at his *samadhi* shrine and from his photographs. Indeed, he fully pervades the inner and outer world, for since such saints have merged themselves in the Self of all, they are omnipresent.

Normally, it is very difficult to get to know Gurus, or to understand them. If someone performs a small miracle, we accept him as a guru. If someone gives a little sermon, we accept him as a guru. If someone gives a mantra or shows a technique of *tantra,* we accept him as a guru. In this way, we accept so many people as gurus that we are cheated of inner satisfaction. Finally, our faith is destroyed and we begin to think that Guruhood itself is hypocrisy. The result is that we stay far away from true Gurus. We get deceived by phony gurus and then despise true Gurus. We set up gurus out of nobodies and get nothing in return. Thus, we end by becoming hostile to a true Master and do him terrible injustice.

The Guru is true, the Guru is perfect, the Guru is simple, direct, and loving. He is the well-wisher of his disciples. He doesn't steal his disciples' money; instead, he takes their ignorance, or nescience. He doesn't seize their wealth and property, but he takes their sins and anxieties. The greatness of the Guru is that he can lead his disciples to the vision of God without severe asceticism. He brings the peace of a cave and the experience of solitude right into people's houses. He shows the spiritual path in the midst of the world. He lets you see the Himalayas in everyday life and Mount Kailasa in meditation. Such Gurus do not advise the wrongful renunciation of property and the wealth of this world but, instead, make us renounce our limited individuality. They are hostile to the limited self, jealous of individuality, and angry with differentiation. They do not make us dry and empty within by telling us to renounce the things of this world, which are created by God.

Blessing him with divine favor, the Guru turns a person's ordinary life, with mother, father, and relatives, into a sacred existence. Then he follows his occupation in society and sees his life as a gift bestowed by God. He performs every action with a mind devoted to God, and as he gains the Guru's grace, he naturally, through meditation, sees the Self shining in his own heart. The Guru bestows the vision of God even while one is living in the world. But a person without a Guru takes an endless array of initiations, dries out his blood in forests and jungles, in caves and in the Himalayas, and exhausts his enthusiasm by torturing himself. He cries and calls out in the name of his fate and *karma.* Finally, when he does not find God, he is left burning with anxiety. "When will I find Him? Who will show me?"

The Guru is a great and miraculous deity. Don't think that a realized Guru is an ordinary person and abandon him; you will understand his greatness only when his full grace descends on you. The Guru elevates his disciples to a high level, shows them their own true nature, merges them with Shiva, and makes them Shiva. The Guru has the uncommon power to transform man completely. He bestows a new life in which there is no old age and no sorrow. He makes us attain perfection in this very world. Just as an owl cannot see by day nor a crow at night, without the grace of a Guru man does not see the world as heaven, but only as sorrow and suffering.

The Guru should be one who has fully realized the mantra and can charge it with conscious force; he should be a master of Shaktipat, possessing great spiritual power. He may be a householder or a renunciant, but he must be able to transmit Shakti. God's power of divine grace should dwell in him completely.

There are many Gurus in the world. In Guruhood there is no differentiation of sex. Parashiva is the Guru and Parashakti Chiti is also the Guru. The Guru is unfathomable. From the viewpoint of knowledge, men and women are the same. They have the same Shakti, the same soul, the same fulfillment. A human being into whom the energy of Consciousness is transmitted is no longer merely a man or a woman. Whatever such a being's external form may be, inwardly, that person is fully the all-pervasive Chiti. Although in everyday life such a one may appear to be male or female, that person's inner being is nothing but Parashiva-Shakti. When the great Kundalini, the mother of yoga, is awakened by the Guru's divine grace, all impurities of the flesh are destroyed and the consciousness of being a man or a woman is burned away in the fire of yoga. Then the Chiti Shakti enters the seven bodily elements and makes them the embodiment of Chiti. When you mix sugar with water, it becomes syrup. When Kundalini is moving within, the body may appear to be made of flesh, but it becomes—and stays— pure Consciousness. When this is the case, who is man and who is woman?

In Gurus, the Chiti Shakti of the Supreme is continually at play. Intoxicated in Shakti's dance, Gurus live enraptured, engulfed in the bliss of love. That beginningless energy, which comes from God and has been flowing until this moment, is still reveling. When She is set in motion in the disciple by the Guru, She burns all his impurities in the fire of yoga. She removes all his layers of ignorance and makes him completely pure. In the end, the disciple himself becomes a Guru.

How should we act toward that venerable supreme Guru who enters his disciple in the form of Chiti? How should we love him? How should we repay his beneficence? O Gurudev! In our impure and everchanging physical bodies, you see neither difference nor nondifference, purity nor impurity, disease nor absence of disease.

Full of grace, you enter us and wash away our sins and uncleanliness. You enter us in the form of Shakti and activate every blood cell and nerve. What sustenance you give; how gracious, how compassionate you are. What friend can there be like the Shakti-bestowing Guru who, through the inner yogic movements, cleans like a washerman all the limbs and organs of the body, both pleasant and unpleasant, who cleanses its nerves clogged with impurities, and takes away all its disorders of phlegm, bile, and wind? Working like servants and laborers, he burns up the inner dirt and incinerates it in the fire of yoga until the body is pure gold. What friend, what lover, what mother, what deity is there like such a Guru? What service can one offer him? Taking no notice of our family or birth, our worth or lack of it, our faults or virtues, he enters into us and accepts us. How can we sing the greatness of such a Guru? Nityananda is everything to Muktananda. His supreme father, his deity, his ecstasy, his meditation, and his *samadhi* is solely Nityananda, beloved Nityananda. "I worship the Sadguru, the beloved Guru"—can I, singing thus, ever repay your bounty? No, Gurudev, you are almighty. Shree Gurudev Ashram* exists only to worship you. Gurudev, you are the breath that flows into me, and I am the breath that flows out. "*So*" is Nityananda; "*ham*" is Muktananda. "*So'ham* Nityananda, *So'ham* Nityananda" —this is how I worship you every day. *Om Namah Shivaya* is the mantra you gave me at my initiation. It is the very form by which you are remembered, Gurudev. You are Shiva:

> *yo guruḥ sa śivaḥ prokto yaḥ śivaḥ sa guruḥ smṛtah*
> *ubhayorantaraṁ nāsti gurorapi śivasya cha*

The Guru is called Shiva, and Shiva is considered to be the Guru. There is no difference between the two—Shiva and the Guru.

So'ham is the meditation mantra you gave, which stabilizes the flow of concentration. When you gave me *So'ham,* you made complete my offering to the sacrificial ritual of my *sadhana.* When I made the final oblation of *So'ham,* I became peaceful, I became satisfied, I

*Former name of Gurudev Siddha Peeth, Swami Muktananda's Ashram in Ganeshpuri, Maharasthra, India.

became *So'ham*. It was not simply the gift of your grace, but you yourself who became *So'ham* and entered within me; you turned my sins into ashes and washed me of my impurity. You turned this bound soul into Shiva and made me your own. O Gurudev! How should I honor you, how should I worship you? I know that I shall always repeat, "*Jaya Gurudev, Jaya Gurudev, Jaya Gurudev.*"

What wonderful fortune it is to have such a Guru as your own Guru, to be initiated by such a Siddha. The word given by him is a conscious mantra. The supreme Guru, full of Chiti, enters the disciple through mantra, through touch, or through look. Therefore, it is no wonder that a disciple can come to full Siddhahood simply by living with such a Guru, by establishing a relationship with him, by living in his ashram, by touching his feet and drinking the water that has been sanctified by them, by eating his *prasad,* by serving him and praising him, by absorbing the vibrations of Chiti that flow from his love-intoxicated state, by contacting the particles of Chiti that come from his clothes and emerge from his incoming and outflowing breath along with the music of *So'ham.*

My respected Gurudev was a great Siddha like this. Rays of divine Consciousness continually flowed from him. Whoever he looked at would rise up, awakened. Great was his glory.

It is said in the *Hatha Yoga Pradipika:*

> *durlabho viṣayatyāgo durlabhaṁ tattvadarshanam*
> *durlabhā sahajāvasthā sadguroḥ karuṇāṁ vinā*

It is difficult to give up sense pleasures, it is difficult to see the Truth, it is difficult to attain the state of *sahaja* (natural *samadhi*) without the compassion of a Sadguru.

Many methods have been given for the attainment of peace in human life; some of these are external, some internal. Many types of spiritual paths have been described in the *Vedas,* in the six schools of philosophy, and in holy books such as the *Ramayana* and *Srimad Bhagavatam.* Only after one pursues these techniques diligently, with self-effort and faith, for a long time, do they bear fruit. No matter which path we resort to or how many types of devotion we practice, it is very difficult to attain the *sahaja* state. The supreme state of absolute unity with God, which is the mark of the *sahaja* state, can be attained only through the Siddha Path. Indeed, it cannot be attained through any other method. This is exactly what the *Yogashikha Upanishad* says:

> *nānāmārgaistu dusprāpyam kaivalyam paramam padam*
> *siddhimārgena labhate nānyathā padmasambhava*

O Brahma, it is very difficult to achieve the state of beatitude through various paths. It can be achieved only through the Siddha Path, and no other.

The Guru, our supreme father, brings us to that state through his initiation. He destroys our sins and unites us with God:

> *dīyate śivasāyujyam kshīyate pāśabandhanam*
> *ato dīksheti kathitā budhaih sachchhāstravedibhih*

The wise men who know the true scriptures say, "That is initiation in which the noose of bondage is destroyed and union with Shiva is bestowed."

When the disciple is initiated, the Guru's Shakti enters him. As a tree exists in the form of a seed, so the Shakti exists in the form of the Guru, and entering the disciple, it induces many types of yogic movements. As the seeker, remembering his beloved Guru, sits for meditation, identifying himself with the Guru and repeating the Guru's mantra, then the Guru in the form of the mantra becomes active within him. These movements, or *kriyas,* are not meaningless or fruitless. It is the Guru's Shakti which works inside in the form of these *kriyas,* producing many different contortions of the body, many kinds of yogic postures, *pranayama,* dances, *mantras,* and *mudras.* If anybody were to see these from the outside, they would look very strange and frightening, but the seeker is not afraid. He experiences from these movements a kind of intoxication, an ecstasy, a lightness of the limbs, a sturdiness of the body. Some of the *kriyas* are a part of Raja Yoga, some of Hatha Yoga, some of Mantra Yoga, and some of Bhakti Yoga, for when the power of the Guru enters the disciple, all these yogas occur spontaneously according to the disciple's needs.

When all four yogas come together to work within the disciple, this is called Siddha Yoga, or Maha Yoga. It is also called Siddha Marga, or the path of the Siddhas, and Siddha Kripa, or the grace of the Siddhas. As time goes by, as his devotion to the Guru grows, as he enters more within the Guru and identifies more with him, the stronger the *kriyas* become and the greater the supernatural experiences such as clairaudience, clairvoyance, and spontaneous yogic postures. Sometimes, however, his progress is slowed down because, through the impurity of his heart, the seeker starts to see attachments, dislikes, and other faults in the Guru. Then he says, "Babaji, I am not getting the *kriyas* I used to have."

I tell him, "You will get them, you will certainly get them, but first reform yourself."

Sometimes my venerable Guru would get angry, and I used to explain it to myself in this way: "Listen, brother, all the actions and works of the Lord are full of the Lord. Whatever they may be, they are sacred. All His actions and works are auspicious and give happiness." You may or may not be aware of it, but is there any difference in the state Lord Krishna bestowed on the *gopis* when He was so pleased with their one-pointed love, which He bestowed on Uddhava and Arjuna by His instruction, and which He forced upon Kamsa and Chanur by slaying them? The state that He gave to Devaki, His mother, is the same state that He gave to Putana, who gave Him poison to drink. He gave it to Devaki out of love and to Putana out of rage, but in essence both are exactly the same.

One of the aspects of God's play is bliss. All works, all actions, and all deeds of the One-without-a-second are of the same essence. In the same way, all the actions of the Guru are the unfolding of Chiti's drama. All these actions are virtuous, all bring progress. By searching for faults in the behavior of such a Guru, the seeker hinders his own *sadhana*. One should never look for bad qualities in Gurus, saints, or Siddhas.

The behavior of Siddhas is very strange, and ordinary people cannot understand it. If you live in the company of saints, you should not criticize them. My Guru would abuse people and even beat them. There was always a reason for this. Such saints possess a divine radiance. Their way is such that they learn from the ignorant and teach

Four
Chiti Kundalini:
The Divine Mother

The tradition of Gurus is very great. It is said that from time immemorial their strength, their power, and the force of their austerities have protected us like a mountain. It is such a Guru who transmits his Shakti into the disciple, pierces the *chakras,* and stabilizes him in the *sahasrara.*

He causes the sublime Chitshakti to descend into the disciple. This is described in the *Pratyabhijnahridayam* thus: *chitiḥ svatantrā viśvasiddhihetuḥ*—"Chiti, by Her own free will, creates the universe." This Chitshakti is no different from Paramashiva, the supreme Lord. She is the ground of the whole process of creation, sustenance, and destruction of the universe.

Chitshakti is completely free. She performs all actions and gives the fruit of all spiritual disciplines. She bestows both worldly fulfillment and liberation; She grants an easy means to happiness. Self-luminous, transcending time, space, and form, She is the creative aspect of Parashiva, the basis of all forms of energy. It is She who gives grace and She who controls it; She is the illuminator of transcendental reality. She is both worldly life and spiritual life. The glory of this supreme Shakti is marvelous. She is the knowledge of the enlightened and the fruit of action of the active. She is the ecstatic state of *bhaktas* and the dynamic Kundalini of yogis. In fact, She is the beauty of the whole world. The whole world is adorned by Chiti. She is Parashiva's supreme Shakti, Chiti, who is exceedingly marvelous, and can be perceived only through great wonderment. The entire functioning of this universe, from worldly to spiritual, is carried on by Chiti.

O Mother Chiti, beloved wife of Parashiva and His dynamic expression, You are His throbbing vibrations. You are the essence of the five elements that compose the universe. You are the sun, the moon, the stars, the planets. O Goddess Kundalini, You are heaven, Vaikuntha, and the nether worlds; You are the three worlds and the four directions. In Your divine existence, You assume the 8,400,000 forms of life—those born of sweat, seed, egg, and womb. You reveal these endless inspirations within Your own being.

You possess infinite modes of being. It is no wonder people become exhausted from investigating the nature of this universe, for the manifestations of Your divine light are endless. You have brought forth this creation, consisting of unity and diversity, within Yourself, but You remain completely detached. You rejoice only in supreme ecstasy. You can be attained through the *Vedas,* through Vedanta, through different scriptures, and mantras.

O Mother Kundalini, You are the blissful Shakti that came from Nityananda. You are yoga and the eight limbs of yoga; You are the essence of *samadhi,* You are the *nirvikalpa* state; You are the almighty sustainer of the human body. O Mother Kundalini, the embodiment of Chiti, You are the pure-souled Guru of all great Gurus. Enthroned on the Guru's seat, in the two-petaled lotus between the eyebrows, You secure for Your disciples what they don't already have and preserve what they already possess. O Yogini Kundalini, You are the supreme deity of spiritual aspirants. O Guru, O abode of love, dynamic energy, You are the grace that came from Nityananda. You are the two-syllabled *So'ham,* his gift to me. Because of You, I am. Mother, You were the consummation of my initiation. With the Blue Pearl as Your vehicle, You appear to my devotees in my form and, through these visions, give them faith.

O beloved Yogashakti, I offer to You my love for my Guru. You are an incomparable bestower of fruits. You hold within Yourself countless powers. Assuming numberless forms, You become the Sita of Rama, the Radha of Krishna, the Lakshmi of Narayana, the Bhavani of Shiva, the yogi's power of yoga, the activating energy within *sadhakas,* and the grace-bestowing power of Gurus in the form of Shaktipat.

You are the Guru. You are the Shakti of those who transmit Shakti. This Mother Shakti, supremely honored, lives in the Guru, becoming the Guru. Therefore, the Guru is neither male nor female. He is only the power of blissful love, absorbed in his own ecstasy. He is the enlightening force of the fully unfolded Kundalini. Chiti Shakti and the Guru are the same. The Guru is in Chiti, and Chiti is in the Guru. The two are absolutely identical.

The Guru is the visible form of Parabrahma; in truth, he is Parabrahma. Moreover, the Guru who projects the divine Chiti into his disciples is not only the Guru, he is the disciple's own beloved life-breath, his own inner Self. Not only that, he himself is the wealth of the disciple's *sadhana* and the goal of his *sadhana.* It is the Guru-principle, the essence of Guruhood, that one attains through *sadhana* —the Guru who has transcended the phenomenal world, who is full of divine ecstasy, full of supreme bliss. There is not the slightest exaggeration in the description of the Guru in the *Guru Gita,* or in Jnaneshwar's song of the Guru's glory in the thirteenth chapter of *Jnaneshwari:* "Compared with the water that has washed the Guru's feet, the elixir of life is an ordinary drink." According to the *Guru Gita,* worship of the Guru is the universal worship:

> *gurureva jagatsarvaṁ brahmāviṣṇuśivātmakam*
> *guroḥ parataraṁ nāsti tasmātsaṁpujayed gurum*
>
> *(Guru Gita, 80)*

The Guru is the whole universe, including Brahma, Vishnu, and Shiva. There is nothing higher than the Guru. Therefore, worship him devotedly.

You will understand the meaning of this only when you have a direct experience of the Guru, who is charged with Chiti. He is all holy places, all gods. What more can I say? The Guru is the all-pervading Brahma taking the form of the universe, and it is this One who enters the disciple in the form of grace, who causes His own divine power of grace to enter into the disciple. To effect this entry is what is called Shaktipat initiation, the true Kriya Yoga, or Guru's grace. Guru's grace is the infusion of the Rudrashakti into the disciple.

When you receive the grace of a Siddha, *sadhana* starts. To some, the experiences of *sadhana* come quickly; to others, after a time. If *sadhana* is taking place inwardly in a subtle form, there may be no conscious awareness of it; nonetheless, the *sadhaka* should keep up his practice with reverence, sincerity, faith, and love. The grace of the Guru is never ineffective. Nature can be reversed, the sun can stop shedding its heat and the moon lose its coolness, water can stop flowing, night can become day and day become night, but once you receive the grace of a Siddha, it never goes to waste. This grace stays with a disciple from birth to birth. No matter which country or world man goes to, his accumulated sins keep searching for the time to bear their fruit, and in the same way, grace given to a disciple follows him until it is time to be activated. So you should keep up your practice with perseverance, enthusiasm, and love.

When the divine power of grace first enters within, it brings sleep, heaviness, and lassitude. Some *sadhakas* fall into a deep sleep. All this is a sign that *sadhana* is going well; there should be no misgivings about this.

It is a good idea to always sit in one place for meditation and, if convenient, to keep a special set of clothes for it. In the place where you meditate, many rays of Chiti gather and settle, and if you meditate in the same place every day, your meditation becomes better and better. I have a meditation room. For a time, I used to meditate there, and later everybody began meditating there. Now meditation comes to everyone who sits in that room, and initiation also occurs there. So the best thing is to meditate in one place. However, if this is not convenient, then meditate anywhere; the beloved Gurudev will certainly bless you.

The human body may look like a lump of flesh, but that's not really what it is. In fact, it is a wonderful creation, composed of 72,000 *nadis,* or channels. These *nadis,* together with the six *chakras* and the nine openings, form a sort of house. It is also sometimes called a town, composed of seven elements. Of the 72,000 *nadis,* a hundred are important; of these hundred, ten are more important; of these ten, three are most important; and of these three, the central channel, called the *sushumna,* is supreme. All activities of life are carried out by the *sushumna,* which extends unbroken from the dwelling place of Parashiva in the *sahasrara* to the site of the Kundalini in the *muladhara.*

Prana is of the utmost importance in the body. When *prana* goes, everything goes, and the body is worth only a few pennies. In fact, the whole universe arises from *prana.* Man arises from *prana;* happiness, energy, perfection, health, travels through other worlds, bearing of children, strength and virility, sickness and anxiety, delusion and madness, beauty, rebirth and liberation—all come from *prana.* *Prana* is Brahma, Shiva, Shakti, and Kundalini. *Prākasaṁvitprāṇe pariṇatā—*"The original, universal Consciousness evolves into *prana.*" Also: *sarvaṁ prāṇe pratiṣṭhitam—*"Everything is established in *prana.*"

The senses of perception and the organs of action are all able to function because of *prana.* Just as the spokes of a chariot wheel are fixed to the hub, so the body, the senses, the mind, and the intellect all depend on *prana.* The *prana* separates into different aspects, which fulfill different functions in the body, so that the body may work in an orderly manner. To carry out its various tasks, this *prana,* full of Chiti, pervades the individual body in five forms: *prana, apana, samana, vyana,* and *udana.* But it is still all one *prana,* one Shakti. It is only to carry out different tasks that it pervades the individual body and the cosmic body in these five different forms.

1. *Prana* works in the heart.

2. *Apana* is the power that works downward. It expels waste matter through the anus and urethra.

3. *Samana* is that which functions equally in all places. Its task is to distribute nourishment from the food we eat to the entire body.

4. *Vyana* is all-pervading. It is that power of movement which is in the many branches of the whole network of the 72,000 *nadis.*

5. *Udana* is that which carries upward. *Udana* is a great friend of the *sadhaka;* through its force, a yogi maintains his celibacy, draws his sexual fluid upward, and becomes an *urdhvareta.* The sexual fluid mingles with *prana* and turns into *prana,* and from its strength, the yogi can acquire complete victory over even a celestial dancer. The source of the power to give Shaktipat is this *urdhvaretas,* the rising of the sexual fluid. It gives energy, strength, radiance, and valor. With the aid of *udana,* a sinful soul migrates to Papaloka, the world of sinners, and a virtuous soul to Punyaloka, the world of the virtuous, before returning to the human world. And it is this *udana* which, when it has become purified through Kriya Yoga, brings the blissful experience of *samadhi.* The *udanashakti* resides in the *sushumna.*

It is the function of these five *pranas* to support life, each through its own particular activities. *Prana* is the most important of the innumerable powers of God. Being the fundamental support of the heart, *prana* ensures that it goes on beating continually and so sustains the body. The individual lives through the work of the *pranashakti.*

The great Shakti Kundalini dwells in the central *nadi, sushumna,* and when awakened by the Guru's grace, is carried by the five *pranas* throughout the body, passing through the 72,000 *nadis.* This Shakti flows into the seven elements, into the particles of blood and other body fluids, and makes the body pure, well-proportioned, clean, and beautiful, giving it luster and radiance. As I have already said, this *pranashakti* does countless tasks. Sometimes, in a seeker who is steadfast and full of devotion to his Guru, it pulsates with its grand, joyous, and ecstatic vibrations in extraordinary ways. At that time he dances, sings, and weeps. Sometimes he will shout, or the different parts of his body will start to move. He may hop like a frog, spin, twist, run in circles, roll on the ground, slap his face, roll his head round and round, adopt different yogic postures and *mudras,* shake, sweat, do the *jalandhara, uddiyana,* or *mula bandhas;* his tongue may be drawn in or up against the palate in the *kechari mudra,* his eyeballs rolling upwards. He may make different sounds; he may roar like a lion or make other animal noises, or he may loudly chant *Om* and other mantras. All these *kriyas* occur spontaneously during meditation. Different kinds of *pranayama*, such as *bhasrika, bhramari, sheetali, sitkari,* or *ujjayi,* happen automatically. There is involuntary *kumbhaka,* or retention of the breath, and as meditation deepens, the *kumbhakas* becomes longer. Occasionally the Shakti will produce some common ailment, which soon clears up, as diseases that have been latent in the body are brought to the surface and expelled. All these movements and activities are possible through the all-knowing and intelligent force of the Guru's grace.

Sometimes a kind of intoxication surges through the *sadhaka.* His head feels heavy and he remains in the sleeplike state of *tandra.* In this state, he often sees visions. He sees Siddhas and lights, he wanders through other worlds—heaven, hell, Pitruloka (the world of the ancestors), and Siddhaloka (the world of the Siddhas)—and he even sees his own Guru. A divine and unparalleled joy rises up in waves from within, currents of happiness flow through all the *nadis,* and in his state of intoxication, the seeker begins to sway to and fro. The whole of creation, even the most ordinary things, seem to him so beautiful and full of love that he feels as if he has been reborn in a new world, as if celestial beauty, delight, and pleasure have incarnated in the mortal world. Realizing how joyous and sweet life is, the *sadhaka* becomes overwhelmed with ecstasy. Love springs forth from his heart and compassion surges for all creatures.

Sometimes the impulses of Shakti are strong, sometimes mild. She may deepen meditation for four days, and then She may reduce its intensity. O *sadhakas,* do not be afraid. Becoming fearless, take refuge in the Guru. Let him be your hope, your trust, your strength. You will naturally become perfect. Always keep yourself disciplined and meditate at a regular time; keep repeating mentally the Name given to you by the Guru.

Nama japa, the repetition of the Name, activates the inner Shakti with great force, for the syllables of the Sanskrit alphabet from "*a*" to "*ksha*" are charged with Kundalini Chiti:

> *akārādikshakārāntā mātrikāvarṇarūpiṇī*
> *yayā sarvamidaṁ vyāptaṁ trailokyaṁ sacharāchāram*

Kundalini, by whom all these three worlds of moveable and immoveable things are pervaded, is of the form of the letters of the alphabet, from "*a*" to "*ksha*".

The Name is God revealed. Repeat the Name, meditate on the Name, chant the Name. Meditate only on the Name.

The main thing is to be constantly aware of whether or not *nama japa* is going on. Repeating the Name increases one's interest in *sadhana* and one's love for the Guru. It gives the skill of science and the experience of love. The Name is the wish-fulfilling jewel, the wish-fulfilling cow, the wish-fulfilling tree.

Truly speaking, the Name is the mantra you have received from the Guru. You should understand it to be the perceptible form of God, and repeat it with complete faith and sincerity. Do not forget that the mantra, the Guru, the Shakti, and yourself are one. It is said that the mantra protects the person who is repeating it: *mantrah mananatrānarūpāḥ.* You should keep repeating the mantra and assimilating it. Keep repeating the mantra which is the blessed gift of a Siddha Guru. The Guru dwells in the mantra in a living form; therefore, keep repeating this conscious Guru-mantra. Sing it with love, meditate on it affectionately, and the Shakti will do Her work with the speed of lightning.

The mantra should be repeated by lovingly coordinating it with the incoming and outgoing breaths. Then, very soon, *kriyas* will take place of their own accord, you will have visions, *sadhana* will come to you naturally. Saint Tukaram says that just by repeating the Name one will understand that which could not be understood, that through the glory of the Name that which was unseen will easily be seen. Repeating the Name brings immense benefits:

> *na kare tem karom yeil ugalem nāmem yā viṭṭhale ekāchiyā*
> *na dise tem disom yeil ugalem nāmem yā viṭṭhale ekāchiyā*
> *alabhya to lābha hoil apāra nāma nirantara mhanatām vāche*

Only by repeating the name of Vitthal, that which cannot be understood will be understood.

Only by repeating the name of Vitthal, that which cannot be seen will be easily seen.

By incessantly repeating the name, one gets benefits which are otherwise unattainable.

You should sit in solitude and repeat the Name with a pure mind. When you contemplate bad thoughts and bad impressions, your mind experiences corresponding states. You have had the experience of thinking lustful thoughts and becoming full of lust. So how long will it take you to become full of the mantra when you have been thinking of the mantra? The Guru has entered you with the mantra. He has spread through your body and will make you like himself. How great is this bounty of the Guru! Again I remind you, keep on repeating the mantra, and through this you will attain the state of meditation.

The Gurushakti, seated in the heart, intensifies and stabilizes meditation. She will certainly bring you some inner experience—a light, a vision, a divine sound—and this will support and deepen your meditation. Meditation is the infallible means of conquering the restlessness of the mind. It is the wish-fulfilling tree which grants whatever you desire, the magnet which draws the power of God. Never underestimate meditation. Meditation is the heart of yoga, the root of *sadhana,* the master key to knowledge, the stream of love, the sacrificial rite that earns the richness of the Guru's grace. Meditation is also one form of the Guru. You will ask how to meditate, on what to meditate, and for how long. These are primary and essential questions. It is said in the *Gita* (13:24): *dhyānenātmani paśyanti kechidātmānam—*"The vision of the Self is obtained through meditation." In the *Shrimad Bhagavatam* it says: *dhyāne dhyāne tadrurūpatā—* "In meditation the *sadhaka* becomes the form of God." Just as a worm becomes a wasp by meditating intensely on a wasp, a *sadhaka,* through meditating on God, becomes like God.

The idea of meditation should not frighten you because, in your daily life, you already perform many kinds of meditation; it simply happens. Your skills and talents are perfected solely through meditation. Without one-pointed attention, is it possible for a doctor to cure a disease, a judge to make his decision, a professor to give a lecture? Without concentration, can one make an apparatus such as radar, cook food, drive a car, keep the rhythm in music, solve mathematical problems? A degree of meditation is required to achieve anything. But in all these things, your meditation is directed toward the world, not toward God. Just as you have occupied your mind with mundane activities, in the same way, to immerse the mind in love for God is meditation. Meditation is not really hard, but it is not so easy either. The full meaning of meditation is: *dhyānam nirviṣayam manaḥ*—"Meditation is a mind free from thoughts." To free the mind from reflection, from thinking, from memory and knowledge, to make the mind not-mind, is the nature of high meditation. Only saints of the highest caliber know this meditation. When the mind becomes empty of thought and becomes one with the Self, this indicates a very high state.

People wonder whether to meditate on the Form or on the Formless aspect of God, but you should not feel any conflict about this. Both meditations give the same results. Saints like Tukaram, Tulsidas, Namdev, Mirabai, and Janabai were devoted to the Form, the personal aspect of God. God came to them in a personal form, but they also realized the Formless. The God with form, or *saguna* aspect, is not imaginary. God's greatness is unlimited. He created this habitable world in the midst of nothingness out of the storehouse of His unlimited power. He alone became the world, manifesting Himself in all its various objects. How can it be difficult for Him, whose names and forms are limitless, to take a form? So *sadhus, sannyasis,* and seekers should not take any part in such controversies. Meditate on what pleases you most. The *saguna,* the Form, and the *nirguna,* the Formless, are both God. Meditate on that which stills your mind, which frees it of restlessness, and brings it into the Self. Do not waste your time wrangling. Meditate on anything. All deities are suitable for meditation, since they all are of the same substance. Through meditation, you should attain the place of supreme peace that is within you. When he arrives at that place, the aspirant forgets all pain and suffering; he becomes whole, he forgets the nightmares of his frustration and inadequacies, and his imaginings about birth and death are destroyed. Arguing is a disease. Man has suffered from so many diseases in his life and repented. Why doesn't he, then, keep away from the disease of controversies about meditation?

Keep your mind empty. When you awake, you experience a few moments when your mind is free of thoughts. You should make your mind peaceful and thought-free like this, so that it becomes no different from the Self. This is progress in meditation.

And let me tell you one more thing. Look upon everything that you see as filled with God. The whole visible world is complete in God.

To have this understanding is a great meditation. It is the true way of seeing and brings liberation from birth and death:

sakalamidamaham cha vāsudevaḥ parama pumān parameshvaraḥ sa ekaḥ
iti matirachalā bhavatyanante hridayagate vraja tāna vihāya dūrāt

(Vishnu Purana, III, 7:32)

> Yamaraj, the lord of death, says to his messengers: "This phenomenal world and I are the one Lord God, Vasudeva. Whoever has an unshakeable feeling for the Lord fixed in the heart, then, O messengers, leave him alone, leave him alone and come away."

What an exalted meditation, what an exalted spirit! Those who meditate on God in the north, the south, the east, the west, in God before and behind, in God above and below, very quickly attain liberation. The *gopis* used to meditate like this; wherever they looked they saw Krishna. For the *gopis* the Yamuna River was Krishna, the bowers and the forests were Krishna, the four directions were Krishna, their husbands were Krishna, their children were Krishna, the cows were Krishna, they were themselves Krishna. Krishna was in their minds, Krishna was in their bodies, Krishna was everywhere. They saw nothing other than Krishna. This kind of meditation is perfect in itself—you don't have to go to a mountain or a cave. This is the meditation that follows knowledge; in this the knowledge of God is vital. It is really true that the whole world is the perfect form of God.

Six

The Importance
of a Siddha's Abode

Many people used to come to Bhagavan Nityananda. They did their *sadhana,* and they all had one wish: to acquire supernatural powers and honor and become Nityananda. Each one would say, "I am so important. I am so big. Nityananda loves me most. He has blessed me particularly; no one else has gotten as much as I have." These irritating and distressing voices were heard among the devotees and led only to increasing jealousy, malice, hatred, hypocrisy, and pretentiousness. And as this sort of thing grew, the meditative ecstasy that had come from Nityananda decreased, and people also started meditating less. It was always: "What did he say? What happened there? What does he know? Who can ever equal me? Even Nityananda listens to what I say; so why should I care about others? Who do you think you are? The Swami should certainly agree with us." Such delusion, and with it the net of transmigration, began to spread. Imagining themselves to be Nityanandas, the devotees became more and more arrogant and conceited, and in this way large obstacles came in their path. In a place where all sins should have been dispelled, where everyone should have been pure and free from wrongdoing, this sickness spread.

A meditating seeker should remember that, just as the mind and heart become purer and more *sattvic* every day through the influence of the Guru's love, these virtues can be diminished through jealousy, envy, and lustful thinking. It is certain that, on the one hand, a man's meditation and his goodness may increase so that he finds peace and heavenly happiness; while on the other hand, internal conflicts may grow, his virtue fall away, his sins steadily multiply, and he may fall deeper into sensuality until he becomes an inhabitant of hell.

People living in an ashram should live carefully. A Siddha's abode is the court of Gurus. It is a center of the blazing and incandescent fire of yoga, which can burn away your sins and make you a master of yoga. But if you spend your time in an ashram without practicing *sadhana,* always indulging in sense pleasures, it will reduce your virtue and make you lifeless.

You should never indulge your personal desires at an ashram. Ashramites should see only their Guru, who is their own true Self, in their fellows so that meditation will deepen day by day. A seeker who comes to an ashram as a devotee should never look for faults in others, for this will only increase his own faults and reduce the power of yoga. Then he will think, "There's no fun here; I'll have to find another ashram." This is a promiscuous tendency. The same thing will happen even if he goes to another ashram. You should not make an ashram a pleasure ground. It's not a center for gossip, a place for college girls and boys to amuse themselves, a tennis club, or a bar that serves whisky and brandy to libertines. If you go to an ashram, do not destroy the Shakti that you have received and fall from the path by behaving irreverently, licentiously, and in any way you like. If you meet people wherever you like and start to gossip, it only leads to slander, doubt, and criticism, and destroys all your attainments in yoga. But if you have faith in the ashram and behave your best there, performing good actions and leading a regulated life, then the inner working of Chiti, the extraordinary experience of Kundalini's play, will soon be yours.

The following incident took place only a short while ago. There was a certain girl who was doing *sadhana* and had reached a very high state of meditation, even though she had been in the Ashram less than a month. Many *mudras* were happening to her spontaneously. One day she suddenly got up from her meditation and came running to me, holding up the middle finger of her right hand. She cried, "Babaji, a snake has bitten me here! Because of that I got up from meditation and have come to you." What a high experience! She had passed through so many stages in such a short time! In Siddha Yoga it is a sure prediction of liberation to be bitten by a snake on the middle finger of the right hand. If even in a dream a practicer of Siddha Yoga is bitten by a snake, that, too, is a sure sign of liberation. But in meditation it is particularly auspicious.

The great knowledge of the Kundalini, filled with supreme energy, is called Siddha Vidya, the science of perfection. This path is called the Siddha Path, and aspirants on this path are called Siddha students. A Siddha *peetha,* the abode of a Siddha, is a place which is charged everywhere with particles of Consciousness. A Kundalini initiation given in a Siddha's abode is called *shambhava* initiation. The *hamsa gayatri* and *So'ham* are its *japa* mantras. The *pranayama* of this path is the repetition of "*so*" on the incoming breath and "*ham*" on the outgoing breath.

All the great saints living in the world of Siddhas protect Siddha *peethas* and Siddha ashrams and ensure the fruitful practice of their yoga. A Siddha *peetha* receives power from the supreme Lord, Shiva, the Lord of Siddhas, and all the yogis and yoginis who are His spiritual descendants. If you are living in a Siddha ashram and practicing meditation according to the way of the Siddhas, you will certainly have visions of the many saints, sages, and yogis living in Siddhaloka. You will receive powers such as hearing the divine inner music and seeing visions of other worlds.

Siddha students, watch carefully. Take good care of the Siddha-shakti spreading throughout your body, the Shakti that has been set in motion by a Siddha. Never look on one another with anger or resentment, or with an eye to see sin or differences. Do not commit any faults, even in dreams. Control your bad habits and don't behave in a way that is contrary to the behavior of Siddhas. Live as a Siddha would live. If you fail to do this, it will harm your *sadhana.*

There is no difference, in terms of blood and bodily fluids or in terms of form and sex, between a father and his son and his son's son, who will be a father in his turn, or between a mother and her daughter and her daughter's daughter, who will be a mother in her turn. In the same way, in terms of the Siddha Science, there is no difference between the beginningless, endless, uncontained, all-knowing and all-powerful supreme Lord Parashiva and all his spiritual descendants of today. Through the Shaktipat initiation, they are all pervaded by the Shakti of the same, supreme Guru, Parashiva, whose nature is

Being, Consciousness and Bliss, invisible, unmoving, and unchanging. The Chiti Shakti, though without beginning, is forever new. In the *Shiva Sutras,* Shiva has called it: *ichchhā shaktirūmā kumārī*—"She is will-power, the ever-young Uma." She is God's own holy will-power, which is His very Self. She is the divine maiden who guides aspirants along the path. She, the majestic Goddess Chiti Shakti, becomes the Shakti of the Guru's grace and dwells completely within Siddha students. For that reason, you should honor any student who has made progress along the Siddha Path, for to honor him is to honor Parashakti. When you insult him or mistreat him, you do wrong, for your behavior is really directed toward the Guru, Parashakti, and Paramashiva. A seeker should have the attitude that the same supreme Shakti which dwells in his revered Guru is in him, because the Shakti that pervades the seeker and the Guru is the same Chiti. Don't insult or speak ill of anyone; don't be condescending or look for faults. Being very careful, understand from within that the supreme Shakti that is in the Guru is in the other person as well as in you. If you don't do this, your *sadhana* and the *prasad* that you had in the form of visions will stop. You will no longer be blessed with clairvoyance and divine visions. You won't attain the various *siddhis.* There is only one way: to make friends with the divine Shakti, with the Shakti of the Guru's grace. Enjoy the company of the *kriyas* that come to you, and then you will have many experiences. Enjoy yourself in these, and remember them with love. Do not diminish the purity of your heart and mind with bad feelings or behavior. Remember that you have to take care of the great Shakti with tremendous discipline.

If a pregnant woman does not watch over her womb with care and vigilance, if she eats immoderately, indulges herself in sense pleasures, and is licentious and corrupt, the child will be aborted or born weak or malformed. If a rich man doesn't guard his wealth, or a good man his virtue, these things are soon lost. In the same way, a seeker who lives without discipline and regularity weakens his Shakti.

You should live in the company of Siddhas, in a Siddha's ashram, with great vigilance. You should not talk aimlessly among yourselves, spread false gossip, or indulge in self-willed behavior, for all this is contrary to the manners of a Siddha. You should not eat anyone's leftover food, nor touch other people unnecessarily. The Chiti is great and exalted; it is supremely holy. Purity of conduct has nothing to do with externals, with feelings of high and low, with untouchability and caste distinctions. The strength of the divine Shakti arises spontaneously in the heart of man, but too much talking and the company of useless people destroys the storehouse of that Shakti.

Many different impulses of Shakti rise and fall throughout the day in the mental world of man. Man is shaped by the actions in which he engages. This is what is meant by the saying, "Actions make the man." Whatever rays of Chitshakti you have consolidated in purehearted meditation should be developed until you reach perfection. You shouldn't stop halfway.

Siddha students in particular should develop this Shakti. It benefits both one's spiritual and worldly life. The following verse describes the fruit of Siddha Yoga:

> *yatrāsti moksho na cha tatra bhogo yatrāsti bhogo na cha*
> *tatra mokshaḥ*
> *śrīsundarīsevanataparāṇām bhogaścha mokshaścha*
> *karasthāvaiva*

Where there is liberation, there are no worldly enjoyments, and where there are sense pleasures, there is no liberation; but when one follows the path of the supremely lovely Kundalini, enjoyment and liberation go hand in hand.

And there is nothing surprising in this. The goddess Bhavani, the primordial Shakti, is the source of the whole world, animate and inanimate. Lord Sri Krishna says (*Gita,* 13:29):

> *prakṛtyaiva cha karmāṇi kriyamāṇāni sarvaśaḥ*
> *yaḥ paśyati tathātmānamakartāram sa paśyati*

He sees who sees that all actions are performed by Nature alone and that the Self is actionless.

Whatever can be perceived—objects, *karmas,* and actions—are all motivated by the supreme Prakriti Bhavani. Whoever sees this, truly sees. Great seers have praised the transcendent blissful Mother, Goddess Chiti, like this: *tvameva sarvajananī mūlaprakritīśvarī*—"Thou art the mother of all, O Goddess—the primordial Nature."

The *Spanda Shastra* says: *iti vā yasya samvittih krīḍātvenākhilaṁ jagat*—"He knows true reality who sees the entire universe as the play of the Parashakti of Parashiva, the universal Consciousness."

This Shakti is the Kundalini, the activating power of *sadhana*. The universe is the manifestation of the same Shakti that is transmitted through Shaktipat by Siddha yogis. Knowing this, seekers should live thoughtfully in an ashram, making sure that the Guru does not become angry and that the Shakti is not weakened. Be watchful. The purer you become, the more divinity you will attain, and as your divinity grows, you will perceive the radiance of the Shakti all around you. The Shakti fills all the trees, creepers, flowers, fruits, birds, and animals inside and outside the Guru's abode, and over it all is cast the graceful eye of the whole company of Siddhas of the Siddha tradition. You should never forget that the spiritual ancestors of the Guru continually watch over the abode of a Siddha.

Seven

Meditation on the Guru

One-pointed meditation on your favorite object is a very important aspect of Siddha Yoga. The Guru has awakened the inner Shakti, given a mantra, and taught you a meditation posture. Get up before sunrise, bathe, and sit quietly for meditation. Face east, or any direction, understanding the direction to be God, become quiet, and sit in the posture. Remember the divine and gracious Shakti. Remember your mantra and synchronize it with the incoming and outgoing breath. Let the mantra fill the mind. If the mind starts to wander, bring it back and concentrate.

Let me tell you another very effective method. One of sage Patanjali's *sutras* reads: *vītarāgaviṣayaṁ vā chittaṁ*—"Let the mind be focused on one who has risen above passion and attachment." To fix your mind on your beloved Guru in meditation is the life-breath of Siddha Yoga, or Kundalini Maha Yoga, the secret of meditation, and the Guru's key to spiritual fulfillment.

A man becomes like the object on which he meditates. He becomes permeated by whatever object he holds in his heart with love. Meditation on a Siddha Guru is very easy because we know our beloved Guru so well. We have been with him often, have traveled with him, have heard him talk about many things. We have heard him speak on yogic *kriyas* and their ecstasy, on exalted truths, on various strange types of *sadhana;* we have heard him tell stories of many saints and holy men.

Everyone knows that whatever is stored in the mind can come before us even when we do not summon it. Once, a young man came to see me. "Babaji," he said, "I am very confused—give me peace. Some time ago, I fell in love with a girl, and since we both liked each other, we decided to get married. However, as we were confirming our decision, she met someone else whom she liked better and married him instead. I am suffering terribly because of this. I can't bear this pain."

I said, "There's nothing to worry about. Just find another girl and marry her."

He replied, "That's all right, but my mind has become possessed by her, and even if I tried a million times, I could not get her out of my mind."

"But why do you remember her like this?" I asked.

"It's not that I remember her," he replied. "The memory of her comes to my mind by itself. Without my doing anything, I see her image moving in front of my eyes."

Isn't that remarkable? He had not worshiped the girl over a long period according to any prescribed ritual; he had not meditated on her, using the seed mantras on each part of his body; he had not received a mantra containing her name from any great Siddha or holy man. Yet her image would not leave the young man's mind. He came to Babaji to ask for a means to get rid of her. These are the consequences of being together. When we set someone in our heart with love, we cannot remove him, even if we try. We say, "Leave my mind!" but he does not leave. This is the fruit of meditation united with love. Then why don't you meditate on your Guru with the same kind of love? He has only to enter your heart and mind once for his image to form and settle there; then he won't leave it, even if you try to make him.

Worldly people constantly repeat this refrain: "Babaji, I try to meditate, but as soon as I sit down, worldly things come before me— the office, the factory, the children. What should I do about it? I just can't meditate."

I answer, "But you certainly are getting meditation. To have your office or factory appear within you is meditation. To see visions of your children is meditation. Aren't you satisfied with the fruits of your meditation? All the things you have loved, thought about, and pursued in your everyday life are now bearing fruit for you. You have visions of your factory and your office and your children; yet you do not consider it meditation. Look brother, I am in the same situation. I meditated on Sadguru Nityananda. I adored the different aspects of my *sadhana.* I embraced and kissed the feet of my dear Gurudev. Now all this continually arises in my heart. 'Gurudev, Gurudev' repeats itself within me even when my mind is not thinking of him. My Guru floods my body; he is in every part of it. He comes to me in dreams and is perfectly real to me."

When the object of your thought begins to vibrate in the heart, you are meditating. As these vibrations continue, the object itself is forgotten. This is a very high level of meditation. It is why the scriptures tell us to think incessantly of the Guru, whose very nature is God. Keep the mind constantly occupied with the highest thoughts. Meditation on the Guru grants wonderful, imperceptible fruit. As *chitta,* or mind, becomes *chaitanya,* or pure Consciousness, you are initiated into the state of supreme bliss. Dear people, think about it! Why have all the great mystics who are established in the Truth urged us to meditate? And why do they ask us to meditate so much? What the sages advise is true and is for the good of all, for the benefit of all, and to give a spiritual character to daily life. They show God in the world and the world in God. The mind is the fundamental means for finding happiness in the world. That is why the sages say, "Meditate, meditate on God. The mind is full of Consciousness. Perceive that."

Man has many means for finding God in his life, and the mind is one of the very highest and most valuable. We can acquire everything in the world, but once the mind goes, it is difficult to get it back. For this reason, Indian culture has evolved different methods to make the mind strong, stable, pure, powerful, and able to grasp Truth for long periods. The different spiritual practices—chanting, mantra repetition, and contemplation of God—are all worship of the mind.

Once, a big industrialist came to see my Gurudev Nityananda. The man had to have two servants, two nurses, and a doctor to look after him because he had become a mental case—lost his mind. Through constantly working his mind, he had made it completely blank. His intellect and thought pulsations had been destroyed and sleep had left him; he had gone mad. Only one thing had gone—his mind—but as a result, he had ceased to exist. He owned many cloth mills, a sugar factory, and other factories, and he had once been a man of great prestige and honor. But because his mind had turned against him, because the lord of his mind had left him, even though he was living he was as though dead. With the aid of his mind alone, with its grace and friendliness, he had run a big concern in India and abroad. Now that his mind had become displeased with him and gone away, now that he was bereft of its company, he had fallen into this pathetic condition. The mind is of the utmost importance; everything is contained in the mind.

Once a foreign aristocrat came to see me and stayed in the Ashram

for a few days. One day he said, "Swamiji, I have no peace of mind.
I am restless, and I cannot sleep properly. Life has no joy for me.
Although I am very rich and have lots of property and prestige, I have
no peace or contentment. I am always full of anxiety. I don't understand why I am like this. Please, show me some way out. I came to
India because I heard meditation is considered very important here.
In Delhi, on my way here, I met a holy woman whose company gave
me much happiness. It was she who told me about you and said I
must meet you. I would like my mind to be steady, peaceful, and
alert. Please show me a method to make it like this."

The mind is very valuable. You should not underestimate it or
think it ordinary. The mind is the light of Consciousness in a contracted form. This is what we find in a *sutra* in the *Pratyabhijnahridayam: chetyasankochinī chittam.* The commentary on it states:
na chittam nāma anyat kinchit api tu saiva bhagavatī tat—"There is
no other thing like the mind, for it is the Goddess Herself." The mind
is the perceptible form of the Goddess, or Chiti Kundalini, and the
whole universe has come into being by means of the mind. Likewise,
the individual lives his life through the agency of the mind. The mind
is one pulsation of Chiti Shakti. God, who is the light of pure Consciousness, is the infinite treasure of this divine power. Just as the
million rays of the sun correspond to and are identical with the sun,
the divine Shakti, which performs endless tasks, is within God and is
not different from God. Although Shakti appears different in Her
many different functions, in reality She is changeless. A sword is
completely actionless in its scabbard; only in battle is it used for
cutting or piercing. In the same way, Chiti becomes the mind so that
the individual soul may experience the fruit of its *karma.*

Don't despise the mind or think of it as an ordinary thing. If
you think uncontrolled, useless, unwholesome thoughts, if you brood
on sin all the time so that you make the mind's state impure, if you get
it involved in argument and counter-argument, you will be doing the
sadhana of a terrible hell. God dwells within you in the form of the
mind, and He brings you the fruit of your actions. Can you think of
any secret action of yours which remains hidden from God? This is
why you should meditate. This is why you should contemplate the
Guru with deep feeling.

The mind bears fruit according to your thoughts. From the mind can come peace, illusion, intelligence, quick-wittedness. The blessing of the mind can make you a poet, an intellectual, an artist, a musician, or a yogi. You can earn a degree with it, or you can attain *samadhi* with it. The mind is the Guru, the mind is the activator of the Shakti, and it is the unchanging, unmodified state of *nirvikalpa.* If the mind is corrupted, it will always cause trouble; it will always spoil whatever you do and ruin your path to liberation. An unclean mind is sheer hell.

Take care of the mind. It is a friend which will bring you happiness. A pure mind is worthy of the Guru's highest love. So meditate with a peaceful mind. God, who lives in your mind, will be quickly pleased and show you His cosmic form in meditation. By the grace of the mind you will easily attain contemplation of the Self. What a precious treasure your mind is! When you own this great and wonderful Chitshakti, why are you sad? Why do you weep? Why do you feel miserable and inferior? Worship the Chitshakti, who lives forever in your mind. Live your daily life always remembering this spiritual principle, which continually vibrates in each impulse of your mind.

Everyone is filled with God in the form of Consciousness. Even while you are in meditation, He will make your everyday life prosperous and happy. Let me give an instance of this. A boy of a very good *brahmin* family used to come regularly to the Ashram with his parents, who were themselves pious and virtuous people. The boy began to meditate spontaneously, and as he meditated, the Chitshakti began to unfold within him. He repeated with great love the mantra he had received. The mantra, since it is charged with the Shakti of Parashiva, the supreme Guru, is not a mantra in the ordinary sense, but a glorious, universal, secret, and divine power in which Parashiva and the Guru live as one. It is alive with Consciousness. It possesses the power of omniscience: *mantrāḥ sarvajnabalaśālinaḥ.* While repeating his mantra, the boy began to have many different experiences. He was just a young boy, but through the great power of the mantra vibrations, he began to acquire in meditation the knowledge of future events from the deity addressed in the mantra.

One day, as his examinations were approaching, the mantra deity appeared to him in meditation and said, "You will be hurt in a car accident and won't be able to take your examination." When the boy told his parents this, they laughed and said, "You just don't want to study; that's why you are making this up." However, three days later it happened as predicted; his right hand was injured in a car accident, and he could not take his examination.

The following week, another surprising thing happened. He had gone with his brothers to play with an airgun on their farm. In the morning, the mantra deity appeared to him while he was in the *tandra* state and warned him, "Your gun wants human blood." He did not think anything of it, and in the evening he again went with his brothers to play with the gun. On their return, the boy put the gun between his knees as he bent over to unlock the door. The gun slipped. One of the boys who was standing next to him tried to catch it and accidentally pressed the trigger. The gun went off into the first boy's chest. The wound, which was near his right lung, was two and a half inches long. However, because he went into meditation, he was not in the least disturbed. He was absolutely calm and still. As he was being taken to the doctor, the mantra deity again appeared before him and told him certain secrets. Even though he was wounded, he noted them down and later gave me what he had written. He was operated on by the doctor. The injury could have been very serious, but Parashiva was protecting him. After the operation, he started to feel pain in his chest. He passed into the *tandra* state. There, a saint appeared to him and passed his hand over the boy's chest. The pain immediately went. From this, you can understand how beneficial and how worthwhile meditation can be in everyday life.

Meditation is not only for spiritual life; it is also a great friend in the world. There is no doubt about this; it is not false. It purifies the mind, so that a student can pass any examination with high marks. As the mind becomes steady, the breath is retained for short periods in *khumbaka*, which strengthens the nerves, improves blood circulation and digestion, and increases one's alertness. Those who meditate every day find that all the various common ailments are overcome. I know many boys and girls who have made great progress as a result of meditation, who have become vibrant, full of life, pure and of very fine character. Through meditation, the mind spontaneously becomes quiet and stable, and the movement of the breath becomes more relaxed. When you find peace within, a new excitement breaks forth in your life.

Nine

My Method of Meditation

It is not necessary to go into a lot of detail about how to meditate. As I have already said, Patanjali's *sutra—vītarāgaviṣayaṁ vā chittam—* is a very good principle for making the mind steady. Meditation on one's Gurudev is the best, the very best, indeed, the supreme way. I practiced many types of *sadhana,* many types of *pranayama,* meditation, mantra, etc.; but in the end, I became absorbed in meditation on my beloved Gurudev. Meditation on the Guru is the basis of all techniques of meditation. When I read in the *Guru Gita:*

> *dhyānamūlaṁ gurormūrtiḥ pūjāmūlaṁ guroḥ padam*
> *mantramūlaṁ gurorvākyaṁ mokshamūlaṁ guroḥ kripā*

> The root of meditation is the Guru's form; the root of worship is the Guru's feet; the root of mantra is the Guru's word; the root of liberation is the Guru's grace.

I discovered my supreme mantra and adopted it with great love. The attitude described in this mantra is higher than all forms of worship and sacrifice. There is a verse from Tukaram, which is itself like a mantra:

> *gurucharaṇiṁ thevitā bhāva āpe āpa bhete deva*
> *mhaṇunī gurusī bhajāve svadhyānāsī āṇāve*
> *deva gurupāsī āhe vāraṁvāra sāṅgūṁ kāye*
> *tukā mhaṇe gurubhajanīṁ deva bhete janīṁ vanīṁ*

In it, Tukaram Maharaj speaks the truth: "Place your faith, love, heart, and devotion at the Guru's feet, and you will easily find God. So worship the Guru, meditatė on the Guru, for God is with the Guru. How often must I say it? Tuka says that when you remember the Guru's name, you can find God in a forest or in a crowd of people." This verse alone became my deity. I based my life on this verse and got the reward, the whole fruit, of making its meaning my own.

I resolved to meditate on my Guru Nityananda. I sat down in the hall at Ganeshpuri, in a back corner where it was quieter and from where I could see Gurudev. I sat for a long time with my gaze fixed on him. His dark body was so beautiful! He had a finely proportioned figure coursing with blood and vitality, a sheen on his body like black crystal, teeth like small pearls, fingers as long as tiger's claws, a belly made strong and firm by spontaneous retention of breath. He wore only a pure, white loin cloth. His right hand was in the *chin mudra* and his left spread open in the *abhaya mudra.* From his throat came the divine sound of "hunh." His head swayed in ecstasy; his body swung to and fro; waves of joy ran from every hair; rays of divine splendor radiated from every part of his body. His laugh scattered light all around him. All this engraved itself on my heart. I stared, unblinkingly, at his beautiful, divine form, and continually discovered a new fascination and magic in it.

He would lie on a wooden bed covered with a warm blanket. Around this bed were piles of biscuit tins, and sweets for children. On either side were two more beds, one loaded with fruit for *prasad* and the other with cloth. I would gaze and gaze at the blessed form of Gurudev, in the midst of all this, this king of yogis, to whom nothing was impossible. People would come and ask him questions, and I would reflect on the answers he gave.

He would swing his lotus feet to and fro, up and down. His large divine eyes, at times only half open, would be filled with ecstasy. Sometimes a smile would come to his lips, signifying inner solidity. His mind was always still, free of all entanglements, of all sense of difference. There was no duality or nonduality, grasping or renunciation, no self or other, no personal or social distinctions, no feeling of religion or no religion. He was always in the intoxicated state beyond thought. Sometimes I would look at him with my eyes wide open, sometimes with them closed. What I saw looking outward I would bring inward in meditation. And so, forever contemplating him, forever meditating on him, I abandoned all my earlier methods of meditation. And as I meditated on him, I began to get a feeling of complete oneness with him. Sometimes I meditated on the various attitudes of his hands and face and body: the *chin mudra,* the reassuring *abhaya mudra*—his hands, moving freely in ecstasy, giving the gesture of benediction. I meditated on his swaying head, on the music of *Om* as he laughed in the intoxicated happiness of total bliss, on his "Aah, aah," which was like a mantra bestowing inner initiation.

Time passed like this. Sometimes I saw him clearly in meditation, sometimes not so clearly. As my meditation deepened, the happiness within me began to grow, and also my courage, my strength, and my radiance. As time went on, I began to feel *gurubhava*, identification with the Guru, in meditation. As I have said, and said repeatedly, meditation on the Guru gives the greatest fruit. This cannot be overemphasized.

My dear Gurudev always knew what was happening in my mind, and sometimes he would make me aware of it in a subtle way. I would watch very attentively all the things he did during his day. He would get up a little before 3:00 in the morning to go to the hot springs for his bath. He would bathe and, on returning, would sit crosslegged and worship himself. He would meditate on himself, and see himself filled with bliss, and would start to laugh. He would hum to himself, talk to himself, listen to himself, and see himself reveling in his own rapture and intoxication. I studied all the different expressions and gestures of Bhagavan Nityananda.

At times I was so completely carried away by this that I would feel, "I am completely Nityananda! I am Nityananda!" In these overwhelming transports, I would feel hidden a great glory, when the deepest feelings of my inner being plumbed many new mystical levels. Sometimes, I felt so mad with the drunkenness of the divine bliss of the Self that the feeling, "I've become perfect, I've become perfect," would surge up from inside me. Sometimes I would study Sri Nityananda's state of mental detachment. He would stay for long periods with his teeth closed, his lips pressed against each other, his eyes half-open, his face solemn, his breath flowing evenly, in this condition of detachment. And I too would concentrate on this state; my eyes would stay half-open, my teeth clenched, my lips pressed together; my breathing would slow down and my mind would become completely steady. And then my head would sway slowly back and forth like Bhagavan Nityananda's, as if my inner and outer condition had become totally identified with Gurudev's own intoxication.

During those days, my feeling of being Muktananda faded, and instead a feeling of being Nityananda welled up inside me. If anyone came near me at these times, or if people I knew started to gossip, I would flare up in anger just like Bhagavan Nityananda. Sometimes, I even abused like him. Two feelings were there at once—that of being Muktananda, and that of being Sri Guru Nityananda—and I was completely aware of them both. When my identification with Nityananda ceased, I would get up from meditation and walk around a little. Then, it was Muktananda who was walking around, and no longer Nityananda; I carried only memories of my earlier identification. When I would remember later that I had abused and shouted at someone, or chased and beaten someone, I would become depressed because of my lack of self-control, and feel remorse.

So I went on, faithfully meditating according to the mantra: *dhyānamūlaṁ gurormūrtiḥ*—"The root of meditation is the Guru's form."

Sometimes while doing this *sadhana* of identification with the Guru, I would get angry. This left me very confused. One day I summoned up my courage and approached Gurudev. I addressed him as "Appa," which means "Baba" in Kannada, my native language. While I spoke, Baba kept making his "hunh" sound. I said, "When I meditate I sometimes get angry with someone and start to abuse him. I feel very ashamed." Gurudev said, "That's not you, not you. It's a *bhava*—a fleeting condition. Aha, that's not you." I found it very difficult to understand what he meant when he said, "That's not you, not you. Aha, that's not you." I spent a week arguing with myself about its meaning, and even then I didn't understand it. So the question was, what should I do? I prayed silently to Bhagavan Nityananda for an answer.

Gurudev Nityananda was the idol of my adoration, the object of my *saguna* worship, my *saguna* meditation, and my *saguna* devotion. Nityananda was my *saguna* deity. I worshiped him as Sita and Rama, Radha and Krishna, Parvati and Shiva, Guru Dattatreya. I saw all these gods as Nityananda. I had no thoughts for any other deities. I wasn't worried by the idea that, "I haven't taken the name of Rama, I haven't worshiped Krishna, I haven't meditated on Shiva." I believed that all gods were contained in my Guru. I firmly believed that to worship the Guru was to worship all deities, that to meditate on the Guru was to meditate on all deities, and that to repeat the Guru's name was to repeat the seventy million mantras. I had earlier visited sixty great saints, including Sri Siddharudha Swami, Sri Zipruanna, Sri Harigiri Baba, Sri Madivala Swami, Athani Shivayogi, and Sri Narsingh Swami and Sri Bapu Mai of Pandharpur, and I had heard the same thing from all of them: "There is no higher path than that of meditation on, obedience and service to, the Guru!" Besides these saints, I had met many *sadhus* and *sannyasis,* including some very highly evolved Vaishnavas, and some naked *avadhutas* who had been living for years in the Himalayas. All of them had said at the end of their discourses that the greatest thing was to meditate on and serve and obey the Guru. I had frequently heard that to lose oneself in the Guru was the best path of all. The Shaiva ascetics whom I had met, who identified themselves with Shiva in their meditation, whose teaching was dedicated to Shiva, and who initiated through Shaktipat, also repeated the same truth: "Go to a Guru. Worship the Guru. Stay with your Guru." I also read the books of many saints. Eknath Maharaj wrote, "Meditate on the Guru." Saint Jnaneshwar said, "The Guru is your mantra, the Guru is your *tantra,* the Guru is your everything." Guru Gorakhnath, Guru Nanak, and Kabir Sahib all sang of the greatness of the Guru. Now, I really believed that meditation on the Guru was the best way of all, and I lived deep in the *saguna* worship of my Guru.

I meditated on Nityananda; I sang of him; I repeated the mantra he gave. After he had bathed in the spring, I drank the water as holy water. Nobody was allowed to go into his kitchen in the afternoon. Even if you begged for his leftover food, you couldn't get any. I found out where his cooks, Kariyanna Shetty and Monappa, threw the leavings when they washed the dishes, and would secretly go and take a few pieces of food, as *prasad.* My mind was filled with joy to be able to eat some of Gurudev's leftover food. I would rub on my body particles of dust from where he had sat. Sometimes I was given the opportunity to massage his body or his feet. While doing all these things, my *saguna* worship, my *saguna* devotion, and my *saguna* meditation grew deeper every day. I never felt hatred toward my Guru, never found fault with him, never argued with other people about him, and never listened to any criticism about him. So my identification with him increased, my faith deepened, and my devotion became stronger and stronger.

Sometimes Bhagavan Nityananda spoke to me, knowing what was on my mind. One evening, when the atmosphere was calm—it was 4:30—I and some others were sitting in the hall, when Gurudev began to speak: "Meditation on the Guru gives you life. Meditation on the Guru is a mysterious meditation . . . complete yoga. All knowledge . . . all knowledge is in meditation on the Guru. The highest worship of him . . . the highest meditation is in *Jnana Sindhu.* Very good book." And then he fell silent.

These words were like a mantra to me. I thought deeply about them; Bhagavan Nityananda's words always had the force of mantra. Pondering what he had said, I went outside toward the hot springs, and there I saw a devotee reading a book in the Kannada language. He said to me, "Swami, I'm reading a book called *Jnana Sindhu.* My mind has become confused by reading it all the time. Let's go and put it near Nityananda Babaji." I said, "All right." We both went in. His name was Krishna Shetty. He placed the book before Babaji. Making his "hunh" sound, Nityananda said to me, "You take it."

I took it as *prasad,* as I took anything that Gurudev gave. If he gave me fruit, I would discard the idea that it was fruit, and eat it with great devotion as a gift of the expanding Shakti; afterward I would meditate for a while. It was in this way that I took the book and raised it to my head. I had already read it twice, but, although it was not new to me, I opened it, thinking of it as a new gift from the Guru. I opened it to the chapter describing the great worship of the primordial Guru; so I went and sat down in a corner of the hall and carefully read this chapter. It was full of significance for me.

The author was a great Siddha and *avadhuta* known as Sri Chidananda Avadhuta, who had directly realized the goddess Bagla-mukhi. He lived on Baglamukhi Mountain, on the bank of the river Tungabhadra, beyond Hampi. I read the chapter on the worship of the primordial Guru three times. It describes a method of meditation on the Guru in which one installs the Guru within oneself, so that one becomes the Guru, and then meditates on him. The book is in the form

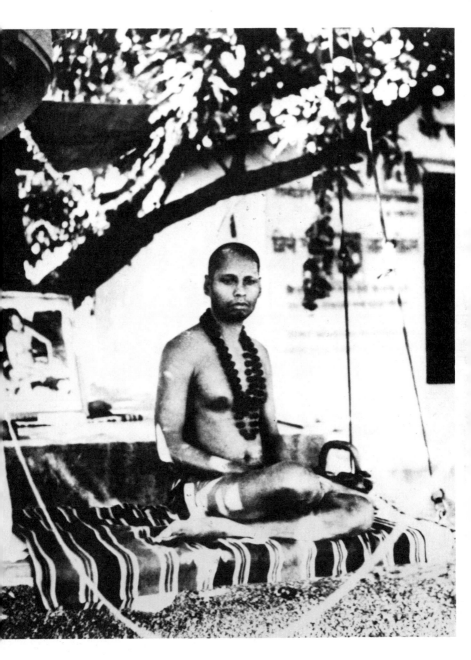

Swami Muktananda under the mango tree in Suki

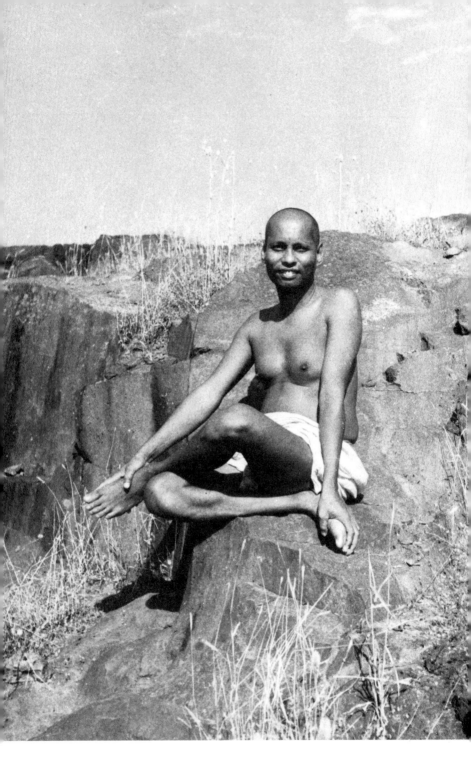

Swami Muktananda at the time of his meeting with
Bhagavan Nityananda

of a dialogue between Parashiva and one of his sons, Karttikeya. Listen carefully, beloved devotees. The chapter starts like this:

"*Atha Śrī Gurudhyānam*—"Now begins the meditation on the Guru." Parashiva said, "O Karttikeya, you are a jewel among devotees to the Guru; great is meditation on the Guru. It is the supreme and secret *sadhana* of the Siddhas. Meditation on the Guru brings both liberation and worldly enjoyment. Furthermore, as one continues to meditate, he eventually becomes the supreme Guru, who is immersed in transcendental bliss and whose essence is transcendental radiance. Karttikeya, the Guru is without beginning or end, even though you can see him in a physical form. His ways cannot be known. The principle of the Guru is the primordial principle, which is of the nature of supreme bliss, which is motionless and yet the root cause of all motion, where all thought ends, where the course of rebirth ceases. It is the ground of the animate and inanimate world, the goal of *Om,* the home of Siddhas. O lover of *gurubhakti,* Karttikeya, it is where all controversy between *nirguna* and *saguna* dissolves, where no one can go without a Guru, and from where there is no return. It is the God of all gods, the support of all, the destiny of all, the true Self of all; such is Sri Gurudev.

"Periodically, he incarnates in the form of a man outwardly and in the form of the Guru inwardly. Through his blessing and his discipline he gives his disciples his own nature and his own state. The highest benefits come from meditating on the image of the Guru, who is the essence of pure Consciousness. O Karttikeya, firm in yoga, that transcendent radiance, which is without attributes, without form, which is the origin of being, is the supreme Guru. All directions, all spaces, all mountains, all forests, all rivers, all oceans, and all great masses of land—everything formed of the five elements—are all the very body of the Guru. From east to west, from north to south, from above to below, from hell to heaven, Kailasa, Vaikuntha, and the final destination of the liberated—all of this is the forever-blissful Guru. He has become all things, but he is separate from them all. He belongs to nothing, and nothing is his.

"The Guru is the supreme goal of the mantra *So'ham,* and the form of *So'ham.* He is the movable and the immovable. He is the microcosm and the macrocosm. He comes, as the human Guru, to

grant his Shakti to his people, his children, his own souls, his dear
devotees. He is the founder of the path of the Siddhas. His mind,
habits, and behavior are in no way ordinary. He is neither a man
nor a woman. He is, simply, the Guru. His body has been tem-
pered in the flames of Kundalini yoga—the seven elements have
become filled with Chiti, and *pranava*—the primordial sound, *Om*
—has become *So'ham,* and plays in his *prana.* All the activities of
the world are the divine play of the Guru.

"You should meditate on the Guru, imagining him to be in
every part of you. O devotee of the Guru, this is the highest
worship. Be still, drive out all the fluctuations of thought, and
make your mind free of all support. Remove all the thoughts from
your mind. Sit down before the Guru. First, bow to him, the
supreme Guru who contains all gods, all mantras, all saints and
sages. Bow to him in all directions, saying, 'Gurudev, you are
everything. You appear as the universe. In whatever form you
may be, I bow to you again and again.' When you have bowed to
him in this way, with your whole mind, O Karttikeya, then meditate on him, understanding him to be perfectly present before you
and behind you, above you and below you—the complete Guru-
principle in all directions. Let your body become filled with him.
Remember that just as cloth is composed of threads, with cloth
present in every thread, so are you in the Guru, and he, in you.
With this kind of vision, see the Guru and yourself as one. A
pitcher is no different from the clay it is made of, and your Guru is
no different from you. This is the understanding you should have.
Now, sit down, become perfectly peaceful, and adopt a meditative
posture. Raise your hands to your head as if it were your Guru's
head and touch your two eyes, your ears, your nose, your tongue,
your neck, your shoulders, imagining that they are all parts of the
Guru. In the same way, touch your chest, your heart, your stomach, your back, your waist, your thighs, your knees, your calves,
your feet, saying over and over, 'This is the Guru's; this is the
Guru's—right down to your toenails. And as you move down your
body, keep repeating in your mind *'Guru Om, Guru Om, Guru Om.'*
You should touch every part again in the same way, repeating the
mantra *Guru Om* until you reach your head. Implant the Guru in
every part of your body, and finally touch your head, saying *'Guru
Om,'* so that you, yourself, are the Guru, you are the mantra, you
are everything, you are in the Guru and the Guru is in you. Con-

centrating on this feeling, begin to mediate. Everyday, meditate in this way: 'The Guru is in me, I am in the Guru'—and do not have any doubts at all about it. Forget yourself as you meditate and repeat *Guru Om*."

Parashiva continues: ". . . O Swami Karttikeya, when you have your bath, you should wash yourself as the form of the Guru, understanding that he lives in every part of your body. When you eat, offer your food to the Guru, saying to yourself, 'The Guru, who dwells in the heart, is enjoying my food.' To bathe the image of the Guru when you bathe yourself; to offer what you eat to him, and to offer all your other actions to him, your benefactor; to recite every day *'Guru Om, Guru Om,'* understanding him to be the giver, the enjoyer, the sacrificer and all the sacrifices—this is the great worship of the Guru."

Again Parashiva says: "O Karttikeya, by worshiping the Guru, a disciple soon becomes the form of the Guru. A person becomes like him of whom he chants, whom he worships, and on whom he meditates. So, the *saguna* discipline of meditating on the Guru, worshiping him, remembering the Guru mantra, and installing him in every hair of the body, quickly brings a great change in the heart of the disciple. Therefore, in solitude, with secret feeling, meditate in your heart on the supreme Guru, becoming the Guru. This is the secret path of the Siddhas, the master key of the Sadgurus, the divine and happy bed that bestows inner peace to the Guru's devotee. It is the ladder to the city of liberation.

"All this will not interest people who are not devoted to the Guru. O Swami Karttikeya, only they on whom the Guru has bestowed his grace can understand these mysteries. Without God's grace, they will not be able to understand and enjoy the worship of the Guru." Having described the glory of the Guru, worship of the Guru, and meditation on the Guru in this way, Lord Shiva departed for Mount Kailasa, and Sri Karttikeya fell deep into meditation on the Guru."

This is the theme of *Jnana Sindhu*, and it was the way in which I was practicing my *sadhana*. I realized that there was a special message in it for me, that I had received an order to do *sadhana* like this, and so that day I did not return home, but stayed near Nityananda in his ashram. Night came. The day's activities were over, and the atmosphere was quiet. Gurudev went to his room. I went to the large hall and sat down, facing east. I began to meditate, carefully following the instructions given by Lord Shiva to Karttikeya in *Jnana Sindhu.* I sat there quietly, and I saw the all-pervading Consciousness as Nityananda. I made myself understand that the five elements, the rivers, oceans, mountains, and caves were the body of Nityananda. I saw the sky as his forehead, the earth as his feet, the four directions as his ears, the sun and moon as his eyes, and thus my meditation on the all-pervasive Nityananda began. As I meditated, my mind became steady. I meditated with the awareness that the whole outside world was completely filled with him. The few thoughts that remained, I directed inward to the contemplation of Nityananda. First of all, I touched my head, thinking of Nityananda. "Nityananda in my head, Nityananda in my skull, my dear Nityananda in my ears, Nityananda in the light of my eyes, Sri Guru Nityananda in my throat, Nityananda in my shoulders, Nityananda in my hands, Baba Nityananda in my fingers, Nityananda—the Self—in my heart, Sri Nityananda in my stomach, Sri Nityananda—the lord of yoga—in my waist, Guru Nityananda in my thighs, Nityananda in my knees, Nityananda in my legs, Nityananda in my feet." In this way I installed him throughout my entire body. As I touched each part, I repeated, *"Guru Om, Guru Om, Guru Om,"* strengthening my meditation on Sri Bhagavan Nityananda. What joy! My heart lightened, its anguish and passion disappeared. Fresh and happy vibrations ran through me, and I was overcome by a rush of ecstasy. When you meditate on ecstatic beings, you become ecstatic yourself. I once heard it sung:

> *safā se milā to safā ho gayā maiṁ*
> *khudī miṭa gai khudā khudā ho gayā maiṁ*

When I realized the pure, I became pure; my ego was no more;
I myself became God.

And so I installed the Guru in every part of my body with deepest love and then became completely lost in worship. It was as if I slept without care on a bed that bestowed happiness, or ate delicacies filled with the six savors. What a divine world I lived in! Becoming absorbed in the enchantment of ecstasy, I joyfully rode in the boat of love on the marvelous ocean of the Guru's bliss, borne along by gusts of cool air, overcome by waves of delight.

Meanwhile, it struck midnight. I had been meditating for three hours, but so far had only finished half the meditation. I started to meditate from the feet upward. I touched my feet and said, "O Guru, please be here. Nityananda in my feet, Nityananda in my knees, Sri Nityananda pervading my thighs, Sri Nityananda in my waist, Bhagavan Nityananda in my back, Sadguru Nityananda in my stomach, Baba Nityananda in my navel, Nityananda in my ribs, transcendent, everblissful Bhagavan Nityananda in the center of the lotus of my heart, Nityananda in the *rudraksha* rosary around my neck, Nityananda in my arms, Guru Nityananda in my throat, Nityananda in my face, Nityananda in my tongue, Nityananda in my nose, Nityananda in my eyes, Nityananda in my forehead, Sri Sadguru Nityananda in the radiance of the *sahasrara* in *brahmarandhra*." In this way, I again meditated on my great Guru Nityananda from my toes to my head. As I continued to meditate, my meditation became concentrated in the heart, and the *prana* became serenely steady there. I felt a stab of pain at the *muladhara* like a bolt of divine lightning. A wave of *prana* ran throughout my body and throbbed in thousands of different nerves. I was lost in meditation.

At 3:00 I heard Niyananda Baba's voice telling me to get up. I did so; I had been immersed in ecstasy. My trance slowly disappeared. Babaji went to bathe in the hot springs. Afterward, I had a bath. Then, again, I fell into the same meditation. It was very fine, and my identification with Nityananda increased all the time. Rays of peace shone within. Daybreak came. Bhagavan Nityananda came outside and sat on his bed. Everyone had his *darshan* from a distance. Generally, I was the last. I bowed before him and stood there. Babaji said, "That's right. That's meditation." He raised a hand in the *chin mudra* and added, "That's real meditation . . . yes . . . oh yes . . . it is . . . includes knowledge, greatness, worship, ecstasy . . . subtle . . . ha . . . that is perfect meditation." As he spoke, he started to sing. I realized that, now, he had really initiated me into meditation.

I considered meditation on the Guru my chosen meditation. I would get up every day at 3:00 a.m., when the world was silent, for this is the time most suited for meditation and singing God's name. I would bathe, and then bow to the four directions, imagining that they were all the same Self. Then I would start meditating on my beloved Guru. It would turn into a divine meditation. Late at night when it was silent, I would meditate again. At both times, I was able to meditate deeply. Sometimes I could not have a bath, so I would wash my hands, feet, face, and tongue, and then sit. After meditation, I would go for a walk. I hung photographs of Siddhas and saints and of Gurudev all around my place of meditation, and it was in the midst of them that I meditated. I never looked upon these pictures as lifeless objects. When I was with Baba, I used to behave with awe, restraint, and purity, and I behaved in the same way in rooms where his pictures were hung. I never sat with my legs outstretched toward them, and in my meditation room, my behavior was always pure, even to the point of walking softly there. This was because rays and particles of Chiti were diffused there, especially during the time of meditation. Moreover, Gurudev is really present wherever his picture is placed and worshiped. Before meditation, I would also invoke all Siddhas, saying, "May all those who through the grace of the Guru have attained God by worshiping the holy feet of the Guru—all those who have been, who are now, and who are yet to come—protect me and bestow their full power upon me."

During this time, I usually kept away from people because each person carries his own particular vibrations. At Kakabhushandi's ashram, the atmosphere for miles around was so filled with the spirit of the divine name that whoever went there, even the thick-headed and insensitive, would automatically become a devotee of the Lord's name, Ram, and start repeating it. In the same way, the surroundings of my supremely revered Guru Nityananda were still, silent, detached, and free of mental agitation. Anyone who came from Bombay would find his mind emptied of thought when he entered the ashram. This was because of the influence of the atmosphere around Gurudev Nityananda. Restless people from Bombay, people of all types, would lose their restlessness once they had bathed in the hot springs and come before Gurudev; they would become calm and still. The majesty of Bhagavan Nityananda's state permeated the surroundings. Under the influence of his perfect stillness, silence, and reticence, everyone sat peacefully, observing discipline. Gurudev was the living ideal of detachment, stillness, freedom from thought, and silence. Sitting in his presence, everyone meditated spontaneously. As I meditated every day, both my enthusiasm and my experiences increased as if my divine spiritual journey were rapidly accelerating.

Part 2

My Meditation Experiences

Generally speaking one should keep secret the divine experiences with which one is blessed by God, but here I want to describe some of them for the benefit of seekers.

One

Initiation

As I have already said, it was my practice to worship and meditate on my Guru. One evening I went to have *darshan* of Bhagavan Nityananda. After *darshan* he would always ask me, "Are you going now?" But today he said nothing, so I stayed on. I spent a very happy night in meditation on my Guru. The morning that followed was the morning of August 15, 1947. What an auspicious day! How full of nectar it was! How divine! What merit and great fortune it brought with it! It was the happiest and most auspicious day of my life, the great day of many births and ages. It was truly holy; yes . . . yes, it was the dawn of the most auspicious of all auspicious days.

The sun had risen slightly in the sky, and the atmosphere was tranquil. I was standing in the corner, to the east, contemplating my Guru. In the opposite corner stood Monappa, Gurudev's cook. In the meditation hall, Gurudev was making little humming sounds in his throat, indicating he was about to get up from his meditation on the Self, and in a little while he came out. He looked a little different than usual; in fact, I had never seen him looking like this before. He had on a beautiful pair of wooden sandals, and as he walked to and fro, to and fro, he was smiling. At one point he went into a corner and began to chant some secret mantras. Then he came in front of me and smiled again. He began to sing. He was wearing a white shawl, and underneath it only a loin cloth and the sandals on his feet. He kept coming and standing in front of me, making his familiar noise of endearment. An hour passed like this.

Then he came near me and touched my body with his. My body was stunned with this new wonder. I stood facing west. Gurudev, his body close to mine, stood opposite. I opened my eyes, and saw Gurudev gazing directly at me, his eyes merging with mine, in the *shambhavi mudra*. My body became numb. I couldn't shut my eyes; I no longer had the power to open or close them. The divine splendor of his eyes completely stilled my own eyes. We stayed like this for a while. Then I heard the divine sound of Gurudev's "hunh." He stepped back a couple of paces, and I partially regained my consciousness. He said, "Take these sandals, put them on." Then he asked, "You'll wear my sandals?" I was amazed, but replied reverently and firmly, "Gurudev, these sandals are not to be worn by my feet. Babaji, they are for me to worship all my life. I'll spread my shawl, and then please be so gracious as to put your feet on it and leave your sandals there."

Gurudev agreed. Making the same humming sounds, he lifted his left foot, and its sandal, and placed it on the edge of my outspread shawl. Then he put his foot down, raised his right foot, and placed the other sandal on the shawl. He stood directly in front of me. He looked into my eyes once more. I watched him very attentively. A ray of light was coming from his pupils, and going right inside me. Its touch was searing, red hot, and its brilliance dazzled my eyes like a high-powered bulb. As this ray flowed from Bhagavan Nityananda's eyes into my own, the very hair on my body rose in wonder, awe, ecstasy and fear. I went on repeating his mantra *Guru Om*, watching the colors of this ray. It was an unbroken stream of divine radiance. Sometimes it was the color of molten gold, sometimes saffron, sometimes a deep blue, more lustrous than a shining star. I stood there, stunned, watching the brilliant rays passing into me. My body was completely motionless. Then Gurudev moved a little and again made his "hunh, hunh." I became conscious again. I bowed my head upon the sandals, wrapped them in the shawl, and prostrated myself on the ground. Then I got up, full of joy.

I spoke softly and tenderly, "Gurudev, what a divine fortune this has been for me! I have received the greatest of all things. Please live in these sandals in all your fullness and let me worship them, even though I don't know the correct way." As I said this, he went over to the west side of the hall and brought some flowers, two bananas, a few incense sticks and a small packet of *kumkum*. He put all this on the

sandals. I began to repeat, "*Guru Om, Guru Om.*" Today I was standing very close to my Baba. He sat down and, in his aphoristic way,
started to speak: "All mantras are one . . . All are *Om. Om Namah
Shivaya Om* should be *Shivo'ham. Shiva, Shiva* should be *Shivo'ham.*
It should be repeated inside. Inside is much better than outside."
Making his "hunh" sound, Babaji went into his room. "Hunh, hunh"
was a mantra signifying many different things. When he turned his
head and made this sound, I would always leave, but this time he gave
no sign, so I remained standing there. He came out from inside with
a blue shawl in his hands, and placed it over me. What wonderful
fortune! From early that morning I had received one blessing after
another. Next he went quickly over to the kitchen where Monappa was
frying *bhajiyas* of green bananas and putting them on a tray. Bhagavan
filled both his hands with these *bhajiyas* and put them on my cloth
with the sandals. Finally, uttering his ecstatic "hunh," he gave me the
signal to leave.

What a great and blessed day, what a sacred day it was! I went
outside, and began to praise my good fortune, "Oh, what merit of mine
has brought this to me? What great deeds have I done that their fruit
should come to me today?"

I was completely overcome with wonder, for I had never thought
that such a thing could happen to me. How could a person like me be
given the Guru's sandals? Nityananda had so many great devotees,
devotees who had been with him for so long. Some were quite old.
Some were big businessmen. Everyone believed himself to be an
advanced and experienced aspirant, and the closest of all to Bhagavan.
I was a new arrival, ordinary and unknown. I had done no special
sadhana and had no special attainment. I had no house, and no business; I was just like a poor man. So, what had happened was just my
extreme good fortune.

My Gurudev was a great *avadhuta.* He would wander through the
world barefooted, never wearing sandals. But today he had worn sandals on his lotus feet, those feet which bestow the knowledge of yoga,
which destroy our sins and are adored by gods and men. He had
walked around, come before me, and raising his lotus feet, given me his
sandals. My anguish had been lifted from me, my sins cut away, the
cycle of birth and death ended, the curtain of ignorance removed.

What a stupendous thing had happened. Usually Nityananda Avadhuta did not bestow his grace in such a direct way; he would instead do it through an apparently meaningless expression or gesture. For him to give me his sandals was something that could never happen. He who never wore sandals had come to me wearing them and, not with his hands, but directly from his feet had placed them in the empty shawl of my poverty. And there was more; he would never look anyone in the face—if he ever looked at anyone he would look from side to side. But on this day he had gazed into my eyes with his own eyes wide open in Parashiva's *shambhavi mudra*, as if he had never seen me before. He had entered me with the divine ray, full of Chiti, which grants all powers. As I watched, I had felt a trembling in my body and tears in my eyes. Stunned, I had, for a moment, experienced stillness and great joy.

In this way, he gave me his divine initiation. Then he beckoned me near. This poor *sadhu* who had come from hundreds of miles away had on this day his first opportunity of being close to Bhagavan. Otherwise, how would a helpless stranger have been able to sit next to Bhagavan in the presence of everyone? This day my special deity, Parashiva, whom they call *ashutosha*—"He who is easily pleased"—had blessed me with the greatest reward for my inadequate Monday fasts and the repetition of his name. It was certainly in keeping with the epithet *ashutosha*. A poet has described the bounty of Lord Shiva just as it turned out for me. He says:

> *dhanya dhanya bholenātha*
> *āpa bānṭa diyā saba jaga eka pala meṁ*
> *tere sama dātā nahīṁ aur kahīṁ jaga meṁ*

O simple-hearted Lord, how blessed You are! You gave away the whole world in a moment; no one in the world gives like You.

Gurudev had sat me next to him, and by giving me the highly charged mantra *Om Namah Shivaya*, by showing me the meaning of *Om*, and by uttering *Shivo'ham*, he had brought me to an awareness of oneness with Shiva. He had shown me the external practice of *Om Namah Shivaya*, the great five-letter mantra of salvation, and then spoken the word

Shivo'ham, which is the form of the inner "I am Shiva" within the heart. In this way he gave me the undying message of Shiva, the immortal Lord. And by saying "All is *Om*" he gave me the insight that all is one Self.

If one who never gives starts to give, then the recipient gets so much that he can take no more. This is what had happened to me. When Bhagavan Nityananda said, "*Shivo'ham* . . . this is how it should be," this great, supreme, and radiant mantra of Parashiva destroyed the innumerable sounds that had been rising in the space within my heart since time without end, making me wander through endless births and rebirths. He had destroyed the endless array of impure feelings, the lust, the anger, the delusion arising from the notion of "I and mine." He had transmitted into my heart that mighty mantra which is entirely Shiva, filled with the light of Consciousness, forever rising, luminous, embodying the truth of "I am perfect," the transcendent word of Shakti. In the flames of his grace, he had burned away the accumulated sins and *karmic* impressions of birth after birth.

Then he had spread a blue shawl over me. Just as great warriors carry shields to protect themselves from the blows, bullets, knives and swords of their enemies, so the holy blue shawl would protect me from anguish, from the touch of sin, from the thieves of delusion and *maya*, and the bandits of attachment and enmity, from disease and mental suffering. And there is more, for he had made himself the priest and offered to me the sandals, flowers, fruit, *kumkum*, and incense. How fortunate I was! I had received sandals for worship consecrated by the priest Nityananda, who was naked and without the conventional signs of a priest. Yes, yes—my destiny was wonderful! And then—something which shows still more clearly the magnificence of his grace—he had gone inside, always making his "hunh" sound, and had brought two handfuls of sizzling hot *bhajiyas* which he had placed on the sandals. The priest was offering cooked food with his own hands, worshiping with the same divine lotus hands, full of Consciousness, that he raised in the *mudra* of fearlessness. At that instant, my mind was flooded with ancient memories, memories of similar worship done in past lives.

As I came out of the hall, I kept raising the sandals to my head. I ate the *bhajiyas* one by one and, again and again, smelt the flowers. The smoothness, the beauty, and the magnificence of the shawl delighted me. My mind, which had earlier been completely still, motionless, and concentrated in the remembrance of my Guru, now became active to the same degree—but there was none of the dryness, the frustration, the frivolity, the anguish, the depression, the stupidity or anxiety that there had been before in the rush of my thoughts. Instead, there was ecstasy, rapture, zeal, enthusiasm. As my thoughts sped past, I looked once more at Gurudev's sandals. I was full of high spirits. I started to sing to myself some lines from the *Gurupāduk-āshtakam:*

jyāchyā kripechā maja lābha jhālā janmāntarīchā bhavatāpa gelā
śrī datta aisā upadeśa kelā visarūṁ kasā mī gurupādukāṁlā

By his grace I was benefited, and the pain of many births was gone. Such was the teaching of Sri Dattatreya; how could I forget the Guru's sandals?

Congratulating myself on my good fortune, and praising Parashiva, my former deity, for his wonderful grace, I slowly made my way homeward. Love for the Guru and a feeling of oneness with him rose within me again and again. And once more I followed the prescribed method for worshiping the Guru and became drunk, repeating, "The Guru is inside, the Guru is outside." I felt waves of emotion, and on these waves I felt my identification with Nityananda grow and grow. Sri Gurudev's sandals were on my head. As I walked, I crossed Gandhi Square, where a small culvert marks the boundary of the present Shree Gurudev Ashram. An *audumbara* tree stands nearby, and as I reached it, my divine *gurubhava* became *brahma bhava*, identification with the Absolute. For a moment I had an intuition of the One in the many, and I lost the ordinary mind that differentiates between the inner and the outer world, that sees the many in the One. I went on repeating *"Guru Om, Guru Om"* with the thought, "The Guru is inside, the Guru is outside," and as I did this, the Vedantic doctrine of Brahman, the Absolute, which I had studied with various teachers, flashed again within me.

I was also blessed by Varuna, the god of rain, because a fine, delicate rain began to fall, and a cool breeze began to blow softly. I repeatedly opened and closed my eyes. When I shut them I saw innumerable clusters of sparkling rays, and millions of tiny twinkling sparks bursting within me. I kept watching them. What a beautiful sight! Those infinitely small sparks were shimmering and coursing through my whole body at an incredible speed. I looked with wonder and awe at their speed and their number. Then I opened my eyes again. Again there were masses of the same, tiny, scintillating, blue sparks coruscating around me. I was overcome with awe and ecstasy. This was something completely new unfolding, not on a screen, but all around me. I was moving so slowly that I did not know whether I was following the road or the road was following me. I stopped near the Gavdevi temple and my face turned spontaneously toward Ganeshpuri. I remembered my beloved Gurudev, and again bowed to him mentally, and then continued walking along the side of the road. The light rain, Varuna's blessing, was still falling. It was marvelous to see the soft drizzle blending with these tender, delicate, blue rays. I walked slowly, remembering in my heart Sri Gurudev, who is the Self of all, and carrying, on my head, his sacred sandals. Even today I can remember that experience of oneness. I still see those tiny blue dots.

Eventually I reached the Vajreshwari temple, which is sacred to the great Shakti, the Mother of yoga, who is known there as Vajra Bhavani. Behind Her temple is a smaller temple, dedicated to Dattatreya, and it was here that I used to stay. I would eat, once a day, with Babasaheb, the chief priest of the Mother's temple. Every day he would give me my meal punctually and with great respect.

I went into the temple and started to worship my Guru's sandals and to meditate. I always used to meditate at night. While at Vajreshwari it had been my routine to go to Ganeshpuri every day—first to bathe, and then to have *darshan* of Gurudev. As I did this, my love, devotion, and faith for my Guru grew and grew.

The temple of the Goddess Vajreshwari is a place of great spiritual force. It is a unique Siddha *peetha*. Many Siddha yogis and great sages lived there in ancient times. According to legend, Lord Rama also visited this place. It is surrounded on all sides by hills, and around it there are a number of hot springs whose waters have the power of healing. There is a small river that flows luminously nearby. Many Siddhas are said to have performed worship there in olden days. I had spent a long time under the kind shelter of the divine Mother Vajra, drinking Her water and eating Her food.

Several days passed. One morning, as I stood before Gurudev having his *darshan*, he gave me some fruit, saying, "Hunh," and then said, "Go." I was still standing. Then he spoke again: "Go . . . to your hut, there . . . at Yeola . . . Yeola . . . stay there, stay . . . knowledge there . . . meditate!" I left, feeling rather sad and worried. But I was completely ready to obey my Guru's commands, for, more than ever before, I understood the importance of the Guru's wish. Obedience to the Guru is itself *tapasya*; itself, *japa*; itself, *sadhana*. It is one's highest duty, and there is nothing more beneficial to a disciple than obedience to the Guru. I believed this with all my heart. Service to the Guru is supreme worship, universal worship. So, with this understanding, that obedience to the Guru is the disciple's foremost duty, I set out for Yeola the next day. In the meantime, Gurudev was to have the Gavdevi temple renovated and three small rooms built there. These, today, form the hall of Shree Gurudev Ashram.

I arrived at Yeola, and the next day I left for Suki, where I had a hut for practicing my *sadhana*. My hut faced north, between two mango trees, one to the east and the other to the west. All three were waiting for me. I installed the sandals of my Guru, ate the fruit he had given me, and sat down to meditate.

Two

My Confused State of Mind

The next day, from early morning on, I was in a very strange state. I was seized by restlessness. My whole body ached and every pore felt as if it were pierced by needles. I don't know why this suddenly happened. Where had my rapture, my ecstasy, gone? My pride and my elation had been taken away, and I was suddenly the same poor, miserable wretch that I had been before meeting Nityananda. My mind was filled with remorse. Where was my earlier intoxication? Alas, what had happened? A whole, new, carefree world of joy had been opened up before me, but now it had completely disappeared. What had happened to the earlier state? Swami Muktananda felt like a ruler gazing out as if in a dream at the ruins of his once-beautiful and beloved city, now destroyed by fate. I came out of my hut and sat down beneath my beloved and unperturbed friend, the mango tree, asking myself again, "What has happened? How did it happen?" This anxiety was burning me up. During the night I had had a series of nightmares, and from the moment I got up I had felt this restlessness. My peace of mind had been destroyed, and all my thoughts were leading me into a deep melancholy. An old friend, Babu Rao Pahalvan, used to come and spend the night with me, but on this day I asked him to go back to his house in Yeola, and so he left.

My state of mind was just the opposite of what it had been before. I was tormented by anxious questions. "Where has the new kingdom of joy I found at Ganeshpuri disappeared?" This anxiety grew in me and caused great anguish. Just as I had felt a surge of bliss before, now I was full of worry and was arguing with myself. My body was sore all over, and my head was hot with the anger, fear, and worry that danced around inside me. It was 11:30 and the landlord came with my lunch. At that time I would have vegetables, millet, *chapatis*, and a little milk. I sat down to lunch, but didn't like the food at all. However, I forced myself to eat half a *chapati* and drink some water, and then I got up and went outside. I sat on the swing that hung from the friend of my *sadhana*, the mango tree. I couldn't bring myself to do anything. Everything I saw around me terrified me. I was a long way from Guru-dev. There was no one I could talk to. I got off the swing and climbed into the friendly mango tree, where I sat peacefully for a few moments; but after a short while, the torture and anguish returned and grew. I cannot write the horrible thoughts that filled my mind, but—it's true—I had them. I was obsessed with impure, hateful, and sinful thoughts.

At 3:00 in the afternoon, the landlord came again, this time with a hot drink. After I finished it, I began to pace up and down outside my hut, from one side of it to the other. People from the nearby villages were arriving to see me, but I did not receive them hospitably or answer their questions properly. I sat in one place after another—in all my favorite places, such as under the mango tree—but only a terrible discontent welcomed me.

My Guru had once told a story that seemed to describe my condition perfectly, and for that reason it came to my mind then. There was once an unlucky, poor, and worthless man. Wherever he went, his poverty and misfortune went with him. If the wretched fellow visited a generous, devout, and rich person in the neighborhood, that virtuous man would become as poor and miserly as his visitor. One day this miserable creature became so full of self-despair that he set off for Mount Kailasa, the abode of Lord Shiva. On the way, he saw a man walking in front of him, so he walked faster and caught up with him. He said, "O brother, where are you going? Let us both go together." The other man turned around, revealing himself to be the epitome of misery and destitution, and replied, "Wretched sir, I cannot go with you, for I am the servant of your fate. I have to go ahead of you so that I can gather destitution, poverty, cruelty, restlessness, mental turmoil, and stupidity, and have them ready to welcome you. That is why I go ahead of you, sir." Gurudev had said that even if an ill-fated man were to go to Kailasa, he would be welcomed by all miseries.

There are some people who arrive at our Ashram in this state. They may be at a Siddha *peetha*, staying with a Siddha, and in the company of the good, but these sad people remain helpless, unhappy, restless, and miserable. Their faces lack luster. They live caught in their distaste. They can't forget Bombay and the dream world of its cinemas and clubs; they constantly remember the ease and comfort of their lives of pleasure. They have only one thought—"When will I get back to Bombay?"—and this thought eats them up.

Muktananda was in the same state as this poor and unfortunate man. I was usually so happy sitting under the mango tree, but now it was disturbing me. Even my dear and good friends from the village of Yeola seemed heartless. At 6:00 Babu Rao came with an old woman who used to come every day at that time and who delighted me with her songs. As soon as she arrived, I said, "Sing the one I like best," and so she began to sing:

> *śevaṭilī pārī tevhāṁ manuṣyajanma*
> *chukalīyā varma pherā paḍe*
> *eka janmīṁ orakhī karā ātmārāma*
> *saṁsāra sugama bhogūṁ nakā*

We are finally reborn as human beings. If we miss our opportunity, the cycle repeats itself. Go deep into your soul now! Don't just indulge in easy living.

This *abhanga* is very moving. It is by Saint Namdev. He also said, "Know the inner Self in this very body. It is only at the last turn of the cycle that you get a human birth. Look after it very carefully or you will have to come again." The old lady sang this beautiful verse with much feeling, but it seemed lifeless to me and I didn't like it.

I asked the old woman to sing another song, this one written by Janabai, Namdev's beloved disciple. This *abhanga* is full of meaning. "Seeing Janabai's great devotion to her Guru, Lord Vitthal went to serve her and do all the tasks her mother-in-law had given her. This is the greatness of devotion to the Guru." Janabai was a great yogini, a great *bhakta* and *jnani*—she was very intelligent and dedicated to her

Guru. In her verses, she always refers to herself as "Nama's Jani" and "Nama's maid," and when she writes like this, she is pledging herself to a full acceptance of her servitude to her Guru. Because he was so pleased with her great dedication and service, Lord Panduranga Himself, who is difficult to attain even for yogis, would come to wash clothes with her, grind flour, clean the house, and sing and talk with her. He was with Janabai day and night. There is nothing surprising about this; such is the miracle of devotion to the Guru. Here is her song of repentance:

> *nāhīṁ kelī tujhī sevā duḥkha vātatase mājhe jivā*
> *nasta pāpīṇa mī hīna nāhīṁ kelem tujhem dhyāna*
> *jem jem duhkha jhālem malā tem tvāṁ sosilem vitthalā*
> *rātraṁdivasa majapāsīṁ darum kāṇḍum lāgalāsī*
> *kshamā karāvī devarāyā dāsī janī lāge pāyāṁ*

Lord, I have not served you at all. So I am full of pain. This sinner has not meditated on You. Even so, Vitthal, what have You not done for me? Out of compassion for Your devotee, You, Yourself, have borne all the suffering that came to me in the world, all the censure and trouble that people have piled upon me. You have stayed with me day and night, and all my hard labor You have hastened to complete for me. You have even ground and pounded grain for me. O Lord, You have suffered great tribulations for me. Lord, forgive me. Namdev's Jani humbly prays to You.

This song always showered nectar onto my heart, but now even this was dry. I could find no joy there, nor any love. Oh, what had happened? How had I fallen into such a bad condition?

I asked the old woman to leave and went inside my hut. I was assailed by all sorts of perverse and defiling emotions. My body started to move, and went on like this in a confused sort of way. The sun set, and Babu lit a lamp and an incense stick. He prepared and burned some *dhup* and performed *arati*. He then took up a tamboura and began to sing some devotional songs. After a time, my breathing changed, becoming disturbed. Sometimes my abdomen would swell with air, after which I would exhale it with great force. Often the breath that I took in would be held inside me. I became more and more frightened.

I went outside, full of confusion and anguish. By now it was about 8:00 at night. There was moonlight, but to me everything seemed dark. Far away in the distance there were strange noises. My mind was sick with fear. I called Babu Rao and said to him, "Babu, go home now. The rhythm of my heart and the state of my mind are not good. I feel sure that I am going to die tonight of heart failure. So go, or people will harass you. I don't think I shall live through this night, and if I do, it will be to go mad. I am losing my mind. Do what I say; go away." He left me with a sad heart.

The night went on, calm and still. The moon's clear, white light diffused over everything. I kept wanting to dance and jump and shout, and this desire grew stronger and stronger. My thoughts became confused, meaningless. My limbs and body got hotter and hotter. My head felt heavy, and every pore in me began to ache. When I breathed out, my breath stopped outside. When I breathed in, it stopped inside. This was terribly painful, and I lost my courage. Something told me that I would die at any moment.

Again I went outside. I saw the whole earth spinning, the sky spinning, the trees spinning. I kept getting up and sitting down, getting up and sitting down. I could not understand what was happening, how it was happening, who was making it happen. I felt drawn toward the mango trees. As I looked in their direction, I saw Gurudev sitting between them, his face turned toward me.

By now it was after 9:00. Someone had seated himself in my eyes and was making me see things. Again I looked at the mango trees. I could see Gurudev there. Then he disappeared. It seemed that I was being controlled by some power which made me do all these things. I no longer had a will of my own. My madness was growing all the time. My intellect was completely unstable. I walked around the mango trees three times, bowed to Gurudev, and went inside my hut.

As I went in, I looked out and saw the sugarcane field on fire. The flames were spreading rapidly. My fear increased every second. I heard hordes of people screaming frightfully, as if it were the end of the world. I looked out of the small window of my hut and saw strange creatures from six to fifty feet tall, neither demons nor demigods, but human in form, dancing naked, their mouths gaping open. Their screeching was horrible and apocalyptic. I was completely conscious, but was watching my madness, which appeared to be real. Then I remembered death.

I sat down on my *asana* and immediately went into the lotus posture. All around me I saw flames spreading. The whole universe was on fire. A burning ocean had burst open and swallowed up the whole earth. An army of ghosts and demons surrounded me. All the while I was locked tight in the lotus posture, my eyes closed, my chin pressed down against my throat so that no air could escape. Then I felt a searing pain in the knot of nerves in the *muladhara*, situated at the base of the spine. My eyes opened. I wanted to run away, but my legs were locked tight in the lotus posture. I felt as if my legs had been nailed down permanently in this position. My arms were completely immobilized. I was quite aware that everything I was seeing was unreal, but I was still surrounded by terror. If I tried to close my eyes, they would immediately open again.

Now, I saw the whole earth covered with the waters of universal dissolution. The world had been destroyed and I alone was left. Only my hut had been saved. Then, from over the water, a moonlike sphere about four feet in diameter came floating in. It stopped in front of me. This radiant, white ball struck against my eyes and then passed inside me. I am writing this just as I saw it. It is not a dream or an allegory, but a scene which actually happened—that sphere came down from the sky and entered me. A second later the bright light penetrated into my *nadis*. My tongue curled up against my palate, and my eyes closed. I saw a dazzling light in my forehead and I was terrified. I was still locked in the lotus posture, and then my head was forced down and glued to the ground.

After a while my eyes opened. I saw a very soft, red light shimmering all around. It was flickering slightly, and from it, sparks spread throughout the universe. As I watched, my legs unlocked, and I returned to body-consciousness. I got up, went outside, looked to the right, and looked to the left. The atmosphere was calm. I was astounded and dazed, recollecting everything that I had seen. I went inside again and closed my eyes. The red light was there, as before. I opened my eyes and went outside again, but there was nothing there.

By now it was far into the night. I tried to sleep, but was unable to. My head was heavy. I stayed in this state until 4:00 and then took a bath. Afterward I sat down in the lotus posture and once again started to meditate on the Guru. As soon as I sat down, my mind became completely indrawn. My body, fixed in lotus posture, began to sway. I felt a pain in the *muladhara*. I beheld a light in the heart space which gladdened my mind, and I began to sway in the inner resonance of the divine sound of *Guru Om*. This meditation went on for an hour and a half, and then a new process began.

I started to make a sound like a camel, which alternated with the roaring of a tiger. I must have roared very loudly, for the people around actually thought that a tiger had gotten into the sugarcane field. The impulse of this *kriya* lasted only a little while. Then I was quiet. When I finished meditation, I got up. My body ached badly, and I was stiff.

Now, back to normal consciousness, I went outside my hut and sat on the swing. The atmosphere was serene. The sun was rising in the east, and in the mango trees, the whole company of birds told me of this with their chirping. The landlord came. He lit some *dhup* in its holder and carried it around the hut; soft clouds of fragrance wafted through the air and permeated the atmosphere outside the meditation hut. He turned to me and asked, "Babaji, what on earth was going on this morning? I found you in meditation. It seemed that a tiger had come. Really, Babaji, I was in the field over there, and for over half an hour I could hear a tiger roaring." He told me all this in a puzzled sort of way.

It was time for my warm drink. This, I usually made in my hut, but today he made it for me. I drank it, wondering what this could all mean. It was true that I had made a noise like a tiger during my meditation, but how could it have carried so far? If I were to speak the truth to anyone, he would have said that I was mad; so I said nothing.

At the time, I had neither heard nor read about such a state. I had only heard pompous talk about Vedanta and explanations of its verses.

I sat quietly on the swing. Babu came early that morning. As he approached, I saw that he was smiling. He was very relieved to see that I was all right, neither dead nor insane. He bowed and sat down opposite me. A dear friend called Patil also came and started to sweep, as he used to every day.

Babu asked, "How are you? You said you would either die or go mad. I prayed to God that neither of these things would happen. I was sure that they wouldn't."

I answered, "What wouldn't happen? Death did come last night. The whole world was on fire. The earth was covered with water. I alone narrowly escaped. Babu, I am in a terrible state. I have gone completely insane. You may not be able to see it from the outside, but, inside, I am crazy." Babu brought out the tamboura and began to sing some verses. I had made a firm rule that no one should come to my meditation hut unless they were going to sit quietly, so it was all very quiet. I listened very carefully. It was a verse from *Shruti-ki-ter:*

> *tū āpa apanī yāda kara phira ātma ko tū prāpta ho*
> *nā janma le mara bhī nahīṁ mata tāpa se santapta ho*
> *jo ātma so paramātma hai tū ātma meṁ santrupta ho*
> *yah mukhya terā kāma hai mata deha meṁ āsakta ho*

Remember your Self, and then attain the Self. Be free from birth and death; don't be tormented by suffering. The Self is God, Paramatma; find peace in the Self—this is your main task; don't be attached to the body.

This verse aroused sublime feelings in me. My body began to twist. I went inside the hut and meditation started. Now, it was not I who meditated; meditation forced itself on me. It came spontaneously; it was in all the joints of my body. All the blood cells in my body were spinning, and *prana* flowed through the *nadis* at an astounding speed. Then, suddenly, a red light came before me with such force that it seemed to have been living inside me. It was two feet tall and shone brightly. I clearly saw myself burning, but I did not feel the heat of the fire on the outside. Every part of my body was emitting loud crackling and popping sounds. I became absorbed in meditation on the light, but at the same time I was completely conscious of what was happening inside me. The red flames of the fiery light soon made me hot inside, and then my great worship of the Guru began. When it was over, my ecstasy waned. I went outside and sat in the swing, beneath my friend the mango tree. Once more, I began to think, "What is it? How did I see it? What did I see?"

I would always reflect on my inner experiences in this way. I would puzzle over them and go back over the movements and visions I had experienced in meditation. I didn't see many people and never touched anyone or sat down with anyone. I always sat alone. Again and again the same ecstasy would arise; my body would ache; I would think about a variety of things and desires and become confused—in this way my days would pass. Babu Rao would come every morning and leave at night. I made a new rule about visitors: no one should come in the morning. There would be only an evening *darshan* and people should stay just a short time. I had this written on a sign and hung it up. All the people of Yeola knew very well my discipline and my nature and accepted this with love and respect, for they and the people of the neighboring villages loved me very much. In Yeola I had grown from youth to manhood, and I had learned Marathi there. Now I was having my second birth near Yeola in the *sadhana* hut at Suki. All the devotees of Yeola used to come for *darshan* every evening, bringing various offerings which were distributed as *prasad*. I was the beloved Baba of all the people of Yeola, young and old. After they had left, I would light some fragrant *dhup* and meditate on and worship my beloved Gurudev. After that I would drink some milk, which came from a nice old cow I had with me at the time.

In meditation I would have all sorts of emotions and feelings and identifications. Sometimes I would see the red light burning and would become completely one with that. Sometimes I felt like a camel, sometimes like a bird. At times I was full of joy; this would be followed by agitation, worry, foul thoughts, and then by worship of the Guru. My meditations passed in this way. After them I would go outside and sit under the mango tree and reflect on the things that had happened in meditation. Then, once again, all sorts of impure thoughts would come to me. I stopped people from coming for *darshan* and touching my feet, for I felt that my mind was impure and my heart full of negativities; I felt dirty inside. I felt that I was ignorant, enveloped in *maya*, and that I should not commit the sin of allowing other people to worship me. The thought came to my mind, "Hey! You yourself are not completely pure. Why do you deceive others by posing as a Baba?" Sometimes I would tell people what went on in my mind, but they wouldn't accept it. They believed that I was just saying these things to

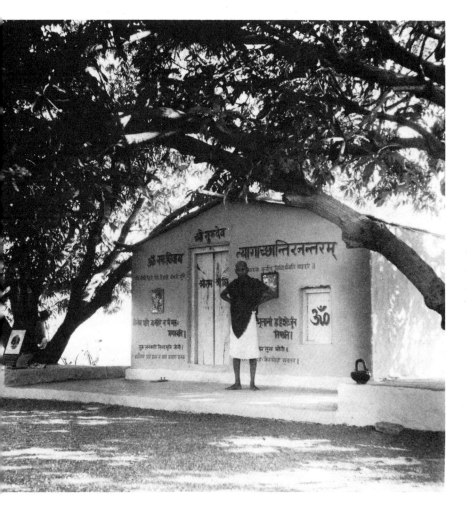

Swami Muktananda in front of his hut at Suki;
the mango tree is on the left

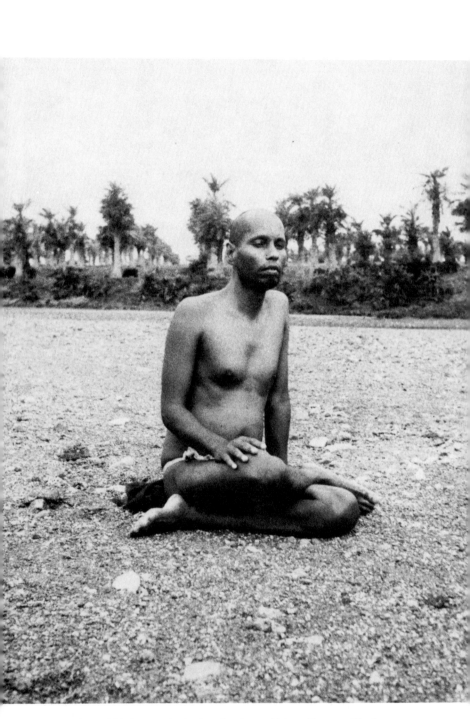

Swami Muktananda during the time of his sadhana at Yeola

hide myself. I would speak like this to rid myself of a nuisance, but people thought that I had received something from Bhagavan Nityananda that I wanted to conceal. As a result, more and more people came every day. Nevertheless, I kept a time every day for meditation in solitude. I had many different experiences. At times I was sad; at times I was happy. Sometimes laughing, sometimes crying, I continued my journey.

Slowly I reduced my contact with people outside, since whenever someone came to see me, we would gossip about all sorts of things, and I would not get good meditation afterward. My mind would be agitated, and this interfered with my meditation. Visions would not come, not even the visions of the lights, and I would get depressed as a result. Besides, these meetings affected my purity and delayed the experiences I was to have in *sadhana*.

At this time, I understood nothing about the various experiences, such as the vision of dissolution and the radiant light, that had come to me on the first day. Only afterward did I learn that they were all part of a process pertaining to Shaktipat. Shaktipat is simply another name for the full grace of the supreme Guru, the blessing of a Siddha, or *shambhava* initiation. People who have experienced it call it the awakening of the Kundalini. The experiences I had had under the mango trees were due to the grace of my Gurudev Nityananda; they were all his *prasad*. If I had understood that all these experiences came from his blessed gifts—from the sandals, the shawl, and his explanation of the secret of the mantras—then they would have taken on a different, joyful aspect. Whatever had happened was due to Nityananda's grace. I realized this later when I went to Nagad and read a little about it in a book.

Our saints, such as Jnaneshwar Maharaj, Saint Tukaram, and Janardan Swami, have described these experiences in their poetry, but in veiled language. The words of these perfected sages and seers are complete and true visions of God for mankind. These men have re-reflected deeply on the individual and universal Self, and in their own *sadhana* they have discovered the Truth and have written about it. Some seekers perceive this Truth while others do not, according to the degree of their worth. However, there are all sorts of experiences that come to devotees of Siddha Yoga which you neither hear nor read about. If you do happen to find such an account, it is usually in a secret language, and you don't find a seeker who has perfected his *sadhana* who can tell you the meaning. For this reason, many aspirants do not understand the wondrous process of this amazing *sadhana*. Their minds become frightened and they give up their practice. Many *sadhakas* have said to me, "Babaji, as soon as I sit for meditation a snake comes and bites me." "Babaji, as soon as I sit for meditation, a naked woman appears, and then I get frightened." "Babaji, during meditation the most terrible thoughts come up." *Sadhakas* have to face many difficulties like this.

Sometimes an aspirant gets frightened by the various movements that come through the grace of the divine Shakti, set in motion by the Lord of Siddha Yoga. He gets confused and gives up his practice. The main reason for this is ignorance about the direction of his *sadhana*. When he gives up his practice due to ignorance, he also makes other people afraid, saying, "This path is not a good one. It will make you lose your mind and make you insane." To take an example, last year a swami saw one of my Siddha students, a good practitioner of *sadhana*, doing some yogic movements. The swami believed himself to have completed his *sadhana*. He sought out my student, took him aside, and said, "Listen, you are making a big blunder. This is not yoga. Brother, I am warning you. I have attained full *samadhi*, and what you are doing has nothing to do with it. You'll either go crazy within a short time or die." Then, even more emphatically, and to frighten him still more, he added, "You will die in a few days, and if this does not happen, it will be no more than a month or two before you go completely insane." The student wrote to me, "Babaji, a swami here is frightening me by giving me all these warnings, and he has told me not to tell anyone what he said."

I left the letter for a few months and then answered as follows: "My dear Siddha student and brother, the time limit is over. Not two, but four months have passed. Your *sadhana* is going very well. You have passed through several stages. You have had the experience that your mind is full of bliss; this is very good. You are getting the fruits of your *sadhana* and are happy. Remember one thing, however, if you ever meet the swami, get a doctor to examine his health and head and read the report carefully. Then say to him, 'O all-knowing Swamiji, you predicted that within two months I would either die or go mad. Neither has happened, and so I can only believe that you, Swamiji, just live off other people and that you accumulate earnings by making a show of your erudition. Even though you are not learned, you speak as though you were learned. I think it is you who is crazy, crazy yourself, crazy for the undiscerning praise of your group of disciples, and crazy for pontificating.'" If such things occur, then man can fall from his *sadhana,* and so a book about such experiences, as well as an experienced Master, are essential.

Day by day my *sadhana* developed and my meditation deepened. The shimmering light I had seen earlier in meditation disappeared and was replaced by a steady red aura, of my own size and shape, which enveloped me inside and outside, and spread right through me. I would see this light for long periods. Millions of tiny rays flashed within it, and as I watched it, I became completely absorbed in meditation. Sometimes my body would shake and swing; at other times it remained motionless. Some movements would take place in my body; different kinds of yogic postures, which I had never done before, would happen very easily. Sometimes I would jump and hop like a frog, and sometimes my limbs would shake violently as though shaken by a deity. And this was what was actually happening; a great deity in the form of my Guru had spread all through me as Chiti, and was shaking me with his inner Shakti.

For the information of *sadhakas*, I quote a verse by Jnaneshwar Maharaj that supports my experiences and shows the sequence in which they occurred:

> *ākāśāchā śeṅḍā kamaṛa nirāreṁ*
> *tyāsī chāra daṛeṁ śobhatātī*
> *auta hāta eka aṅguṣṭa dusareṁ*
> *parvārdha masureṁ pramāṇa heṁ*
> *rakta ṣveta śāma nilavarṇa āhe*
> *pīta keśara he mājīṁ tetheṁ*

tayāchā makaranda svarūpa tem śuddha
brahmādikā bodha hāchī jhālā
jnānadeva mhaṇe nivrittī prasādem
nijarūpa govinde janīm pāhatām

Sri Jnaneshwar, lord of yoga, the true soul of all Gurus, emperor of the enlightened, and king of divine lovers, who is worthy of our reverent daily remembrance, has described in this verse all the stages of Siddha Yoga, the state that comes from receiving the grace of the Guru, and the subtle visions that may come during that period of *sadhana* when one has experiences that are subtler than the subtlest. It is a complete testimony of the highest truth. It is a mantra, a guide for all *sadhakas* on the spiritual path.

The full meaning of the verse is as follows: "The whole body is like a lotus which has four petals of four kinds, colors, and sizes. Each of these has its own significance. The first is the gross body; its color is red. The second petal is the subtle body, in which we sleep and experience dreams. It is the size of a thumb, and its color is white. The third petal is the causal body. It is the size of the tip of the third finger, and its color is black. The fourth petal is the supracausal body, which is as small as a sesame seed. Its color is blue. This last body is of the greatest importance. It is very brilliant; it is the foundation of *sadhana*; it is the highest inner vision."

The power of the Guru's grace enters the disciple's body in a subtle form and does many great things. Just as a tiny spark falls into grass and in no time becomes a blazing fire, so the Chiti Shakti enters the Siddha student and, uniting with his Shakti, performs many functions. Its first task involves the red petal, which is eight hands high, the same length as the human body. This body is the vehicle for experiencing happiness and pain, and it is through this body that sins are committed or good deeds performed. Through it, the individual follows the path of righteousness and liberation. Equipped with five senses of perception and five organs of action, five *pranas*, and four psychic instruments, the individual soul inhabits the eyes and undergoes experiences in the gross body. The red body is the experiencer in the waking state. Without this body, the existence of the *jivatma*, the individual soul, would not be known. The individual soul in this body is known as *vishva*, and is represented by "*A*," the first letter in *Aum*.

When the Kundalini Shakti is awakened, many different movements, or *kriyas*, take place in the gross body. These *kriyas* are not meaningless; they destroy sicknesses and purify the *nadis*. These *kriyas* are different from the movements of the other bodies. Usually, many different *kriyas* take place, continuing over a long period. When meditation on the red light begins, one has various experiences each day, and through these experiences one's concentration steadily increases and the *nadis* become purified.

THE FOUR BODIES OF THE INDIVIDUAL SOUL

BODY:	GROSS	SUBTLE	CAUSAL	SUPRA-CAUSAL
SIZE:	3½ LENGTHS (Full Body Size)	THUMB	FINGER-TIP	LENTIL SEED
COLOUR:	RED	WHITE	BLACK	BLUE
STATE:	WAKING	DREAM	SLEEP	TURIYA (Transcendent)
NAME:	VISHVA	TAIJASA	PRAJNA	TURYA
SEAT:	EYES	THROAT	HEART	SAHASRAR
SYMBOL:	'A'	'U'	'M'	CRESCENT

At this time I did not know that I had received the sacred Shaktipat.
For two consecutive days I saw a number of different lights along with
the red light. I was fully conscious of everything that was happening
in meditation, and I was also happy. As I watched the lights I would
see naked men and children, cows, and herds of splendid war horses.
Sometimes I would see the images of the deities in the temples in neighboring villages. I meditated without fail every morning and every
evening for two hours or sometimes longer, and I meditated with great
love. Sometimes a very pure intoxication would come over me—what
ecstasy that was!—but I did not have the strength to bear it; as I became
absorbed in that intoxication, I would fall asleep.

While I was sitting, I would enter Tandraloka, the state of *tandra*.
In this state I would seem to be sleeping, but it was not my ordinary
sleep state, for in the sleep from which I awoke every morning, I did
not have the same rapturous experiences nor did I have any visions.
But the visions I saw in the sleep of *tandra*-meditation were quite
genuine. I would see something that was going to happen, and it would
actually happen. I would see somebody come, and then he would
come. In *tandra* I would go to some other world and stay there for
some time. Over and over again I gave myself up to the tremendous
ecstasy that arose from all this. After meditation I would spend the
whole day full of joy and delight and love, and all my body's weak-
nesses would leave me.

The state of *tandra* is different from sleep and dreaming; it is the state of omniscience. All visions that are seen in this state turn out to be true. Through my own experiences I have become convinced that our ancient sages and seers were actually clairvoyant and all-knowing.

After I arose from *tandra* I would go and sit on my swing under the mango tree and think about how I had entered this *tandra* state and about the worlds I had just visited. The state of *tandra* would come to me of its own accord, out of the complete freedom and inspiration of the Shakti.

Every day I had meditation like that. Sometimes my body would writhe and twist like a snake's, and a hissing sound would come from inside me. There was a very fine cobra living near my hut. It was old and very wise. I saw it, if not every day, at least once or twice a week, and it stayed there for a long time. Other people also saw it sometimes. I was very fond of it. I have been told that wherever someone is practicing yoga *sadhana* there is always some sign of Shiva, the Lord of Yoga. The cobra is a definite sign of Paramashiva. On the days when I saw him, my meditation was particularly joyful. I used to call him "Baba Nageshwara." Cobras have psychic instruments and show great respect for holy men. I was always very fortunate. Besides his presence, there were many people in Suki who were ready to serve me in whatever way my *sadhana* required.

I decided to eat less and changed my diet to just some rice and one or two simple vegetable dishes. At night I was happy with just a little milk. During meditation bad feelings were coming up as well as good ones—unnecessary anger, temptations, cruelty. I don't know why they came to me. I would suddenly remember someone who had been unkind to me ten years before, and my mind would be filled with anger against him. When the feeling had passed, I would feel remorse and shame.

Meditation at the red stage, the stage of the red aura, is meditation in the gross body. As the red stage progressed, my body gradually became thinner and lighter. I was losing fat without any medicines. Sometimes I could feel a force moving through the nerves of my hands. Sometimes *prana* would flow very quickly along the nerves of the lower part of my back. I couldn't understand what was working so dynamically inside me. Sometimes my neck moved so violently that it made loud cracking sounds, and I became frightened. Was it because of some wind imbalance? I had many astonishing movements like this. Sometimes my neck would roll my head around so vigorously that it would bend right below my shoulders so that I could see my back. When the intensity lessened, I became peaceful again. But because I did not understand these *kriyas*, I was always worried and afraid. Later, however, I learned that this was a Hatha Yogic process effected by the Goddess Kundalini in order for Her to move up through the spinal column into the *sahasrara*. Sometimes as my neck rotated, my chin would get fixed in the jugular notch below the throat. This is a divine Hatha Yogic contraction or lock, which is called the *jalandhara bandha*. As this *bandha* took place there was another movement below—my anus would be automatically drawn in and then released.

In meditation I would see the whole complex of *nadis* in my body and the *prana* moving in them. The circulation of the *prana* in the *nadis* is obstructed by impurities caused by the wrong kind of food and indulgence in pleasure. I realized after my experiences of Siddha Yoga *kriyas* that this obstruction is the cause of sickness and old age.

The beloved Sri Kundalini, who is the very soul of my Gurudev, took upon Herself many forms to spread throughout my body and to bring about these physical *kriyas*. Sometimes She would sit me in the lotus posture and put my head on the ground in front of me, holding me for long periods in the *yoga mudra*. All these movements happened spontaneously; I was learning about yoga through inner inspiration. Sometimes my head would fall back. Sometimes my eyes were focused on the tip of my nose, and in this position I breathed forcefully in and out, in the style of a blacksmith's bellows. Sometimes during this movement all the breath was expelled. Later, I learned that this was a variety of *bhasrika*, a kind of *pranayama* that eliminates stomach sickness and completely purifies the *prana*.

Five

Sexual Excitement

Every day brought new *kriyas* and new experiences. One day, my body and senses became possessed by sexual desire. I don't know why the one thing that should not have happened to me did happen. I had no wish for any sensual pleasure. I had seen the world, people of all types and all conditions; I had seen everyone from kings to commoners, and I had seen what happened to them in the end. In Ganeshpuri, all sorts of people would come to visit my Gurudev, for a saint belongs to everyone. There would be businessmen, rich men, great artists, famous movie stars, singers, public speakers, top government officials. They all had some problem that they wanted to talk about. And whatever else they had, there was one thing they all lacked—a healthy body. They would say, "Bhagavan, I've got everything I want, but my heart is no good. My sense organs are weak. The doctors won't let me travel or eat a full meal." "Babaji, my stomach hurts terribly. I've spent thousands of *rupees* on it in England and America, but the disease still remains." "Bhagavan, I've got everything, but I can't digest anything. I can't sleep. I've spent two hundred thousand *rupees* on treatment." One person would have a bad ear; another, a bad eye. Everybody brought his troubles and miseries to Bhagavan Nityananda. Each one was poor in something, was lacking something, and wept pitifully. One was rich, but poor in health. Another was healthy, but had no money. A third was illiterate—poor in knowledge. A fourth was ugly—poor in beauty. This one had no husband; that one had no wife; another had no son. In this way, whoever came brought his own poverty and would tell of his own pathetic condition. I listened quietly to all of it and wondered what lesson and benefit could be derived from all these people. To tell the truth, my condition was also like theirs—poor in *sadhana*, Self-knowledge, and realization. I would look closely at them —pallid, restless, sick—rich, but still not satisfied. There was no strength and energy in them, only more and more new sicknesses. I realized that the cause of it all was waste of sexual fluid, sensuality, and most of all, irregular living. Man thinks he is fortunate if he can experience sensual enjoyments. He deludes himself by thinking that he is going to enjoy pleasures, but doesn't realize that his pleasures will, in fact, enjoy him. In the end he becomes the victim of all sorts of sicknesses. People are still complaining of this—I meet people who suffer from one new sickness after another. At that time, after seeing the state of all the people who came to meet Babaji, I had only one desire, and that was for *sadhana*.

When I knew all this, why did I have to be plagued by sexual desire? I was meditating in my hut at Suki, and in meditation I was seeing the red light. I was happy. Then, in the middle of my meditation, came a *kriya* that was utterly humiliating. Why should such a thing happen to me? I should not even be talking about it here. Anybody who heard me talking about it would say that I was being indiscreet. Most people would say, "That's what *sannyasis* are like nowadays; they just live off other people. A householder's life is better, since you can enjoy everything and still be spiritual."

Now I shall tell my shameful story. My dear mothers, my dear sisters—you are all different forms of Shakti. Please don't feel angry with me because of my hateful story. Give me your blessings, and think about my motive for telling it. My dear readers and other *sadhakas*—try to understand why I have to write this.

As I sat in meditation, I would see the divine red light. Intense feelings would arise inside me, and I would sway or jump or shake or move around. I would do the great worship of my Guru, meditating on the Guru inside me and on the Guru outside me, repeating "*Guru Om, Guru Om*," and becoming blissfully absorbed in identification with my Guru.

Then a ruinous kind of meditation came to me—a sensual meditation, a meditation of desire. How disgusting it was! I saw the red light, but its color changed. It was my size and was shining like the soft rays of the morning light in the east. All the love and intoxication I had felt in meditation left me. My identification with Nityananda went away. My Guru worship and the mantra *Guru Om, Guru Om* disappeared. Instead, in their place came a powerful sexual desire. Who knows where it had been hidden all this time? It completely possessed me. I was amazed at the uncontrollable strength in my sex organ, which was, after all, only a lump of flesh. It became intensely agitated.

Alas, alas. This was far worse than the experience of the end of the world that I had had on the first day. Now, everything was directed outward, toward sex, sex, sex. I could think of nothing but sex! My whole body boiled with lust, and I cannot describe the agony of my sexual organ. I tried to explain it to myself in some way, but I couldn't. The only good thing was that I was able to keep firmly in the lotus posture; that was as steady as ever.

When I shut my eyes, I saw, right in front of me, a beautiful naked girl inside the red light. Even though I didn't want to see her, she appeared. Full of fear and remorse, I opened my eyes. I still saw the divine red light. Within it, Jagadamba, the naked girl, still stood. If I shut my eyes, she was there, and if I opened them, she was there. What could I do? Whom could I tell about my embarrassing situation? It was all being forced on me against my will. How powerful was the craving of my sex organ! Only Bhagavan Nityananda, or a *sadhaka* who had gone through the same experiences, could understand. I was overcome with remorse and could not meditate anymore, because I would remember this sexual desire. I felt frightened, ashamed, discontented. It started to affect my brain. I brooded, and my anxiety grew. I thought, "This disaster is the result of some terrible sin."

I went outside and sat on the swing, still thinking the same thoughts, that added to my remorse. "What is this weakness of mine? Oh! What shall I do now?"

Afternoon came, and I meditated a little, but the same naked woman appeared. At times she laughed; at times she smiled; at times she stood; at times she sat. I could not bear to see her anymore. The earlier visions, which had calmed and purified my senses, which had brought a rush of love to my heart so that I drank supreme ecstasy, had all disappeared, leaving their very opposite. My sex organ would become stimulated, excited, powerful. Other shameful things would happen, which would make me get up quickly from meditation.

At night, when I meditated, the same things would happen. First, meditation, then the aura of the red goddess would appear. My mind would be gladdened, my heart filled with joy; there would be Guru worship with deep faith and reverence, a strong feeling of identification with my Guru, complete absorption in him. Then the light would abruptly change, and the same naked female would pursue me. She would dance in front of me for awhile, moving her body suggestively, and jump and turn around. If I opened my eyes, I would still see her. I was losing control of my senses. I was afraid that something irrevocable would happen.

I decided to make my body weaker and thinner, so I stopped drinking milk and reduced my intake of water. I could not sleep at night because of the turmoil in my mind. I would remember Ganeshpuri and think for a long time about Bhagavan Nityananda. I would bow to him and fall asleep. In the mornings I got up early. Sometimes I bathed at 3:00; otherwise I would just wash my hands and feet. Then I would smear holy ash, charged with mantras, on my body and sit down to meditate. As soon as I sat down, my meditation would start with full force. The red aura of my own size would arise immediately. I performed the full worship of my Guru. Almost immediately I was deep in *samadhi*, and then, suddenly, full of sexual desire. The naked woman pursued me and stood before me. She tortured me more and more. She was goading me for one thing: she wanted to break my sacred vow of celibacy. God knows where she came from; no one had invited her.

She did not ask anything from me. She simply ruined my meditation, disturbed my sex organ, and did everything she could to make me break my vow. What had happened to me? It was one of the most painful times in my life; never before had I met with such trouble.

After a short time my meditation stopped. I went outside and sat quietly on my usual bench. "What shall I do?" I wondered. "How can I save myself from this terrible disaster?" My suffering, worry, and slight madness increased. I sat there deep in depression. I began to feel afraid of all women. My courage had waned. I was afraid that I might indulge in wanton behavior. I kept thinking of all the *sadhakas* of former times who had fallen from yoga, deviated from the path, and destroyed all their good *karma*. I remembered the stories of Ajamila, Surdas, and even Saint Tulsidas, and wept. The overwhelming power of Kamaraja, the king of lust, terrified me. I had made my sexual organ lifeless and useless by the mastery of *siddhasana*, but even so this dead sense had come to life. It was amazing, it was a tremendous surprise. I remembered the old story of what Parashara had done in his boat. Reflecting on many such incidents, I felt greatly troubled. Even during my afternoon meditation, the agitation of my sexual organ increased.

I asked the landlord, whose wife used to cook my food, to have it prepared by a man rather than a woman. I started to eat only a little rice. I stopped eating vegetables; I would get up from my meals with my stomach half full and have some water.

One day, as I walked outside, I thought, "What can I do to save myself from all this? Who can tell me what to do? When my sex organ comes back to life after I have rendered it inert through *siddhasana*, what can I set out to do with any hope?" As I thought, I became increasingly unhappy, increasingly miserable and distraught. It became late afternoon. About twenty miles away, in Baijapur, there lived a Siddha called Harigiri Baba, of whom I was very fond. I kept thinking of him. He might be able to save me. Otherwise, I could expect a terrible fate the next day. These things were too secret to tell anyone else, so I wept and wept. My head was heavy and deaf from weeping. Night fell. I didn't eat or drink anything. After a while Babu Rao arrived. He spoke to me, but I didn't hear. I started saying to myself, "O my mind, don't get upset."

I started my evening meditation as usual. It was a good meditation. The red aura, the good fortune of yogis, arose, giving out a radiance of numberless small saffron-colored sparks that glittered before my eyes. I began the worship of Gurudev and became immersed in identification with him. I experienced a number of different *mudras* and states, and then I heard an indistinct sound within me. I felt very happy. Then, at this moment of happiness, the goddess appeared, naked except for the jewels that adorned her. I looked at her and then opened my eyes, but I could still see her. My earlier joy was destroyed and my posture spoiled.

Slowly, I got up and went outside. I sat down under the mango tree and waited. Midnight came, and I went inside to sleep, but my mind was not at peace as it had been on previous days. It became mad and deluded. I couldn't sleep. I tossed and turned until 3:00, when finally I closed my eyes for a bit. Then I got up, bathed, and sat for meditation. I felt bad. I was not ill, but was restless and disturbed. I bowed to the four directions and propitiated all the gods. Then I sat for meditation. It came very quickly, and soon I got into the *tandra* state. The red aura glimmered everywhere, outside and inside me. My body moved in some *kriyas*. My throat closed for a short time in *jalandhara bandha*, and at the same time I adopted the *mula bandha*. Very soon these locks were released. I heard an indistinct blurring sound inside me, and as I listened to it, my mind became focused on it. It was bliss—nothing but bliss. Then an oval-shaped white light, a little larger than a large plum, appeared with the red light and quickly disappeared again. Encouraged by this new experience, I began lovingly to perform my Guru worship and Guru meditation. I remembered having propitiated all the gods and goddesses, and thought that this was why my meditation was so good. Suddenly, there was a change in the tone of the red light, though it was still red. Then what? The woman came. It was too much. I was confounded.

This time she was beautifully adorned and extraordinarily attractive. My mind became very restless. My sexual organ became agitated with great force. I opened my eyes. I still saw her outside. I closed my eyes and saw her inside. Tearing my loincloth, my generative organ dug forcibly into my navel, where it remained for some time. Who was raping me like this? I was completely conscious, and my meditation stopped. For meditation I used to wear a muslin loincloth, leaving the rest of my body completely naked. When I saw that the loincloth was torn, I got very angry, so angry that my mind became clouded. It was 5:00 in the morning. I got up, put on a new loincloth, and went outside. I resolved to go somewhere where no one knew me. My mind was in a terrible state. I sat down, thinking, "Now I'll either go mad or do something terrible." I remembered my *karma* and was very worried.

As I was sitting quietly on the swing, morning came. I was thinking, "Where shall I go? This is no good. It isn't *sadhana*, nor is it God's grace. It's the fruit of my previous sins." As I was thinking all this, *tandra* came upon me, so I went inside and again sat for meditation. It started immediately. Now I began to roar like a lion. My tongue came right out of my mouth. I went on roaring for forty-five minutes, getting more and more frightened. This time there was no sexual desire, but it seemed that I was to be saved from one danger only to meet another. There is a saying, "Fall out of the sky and get stuck in a palm tree," and that was how I felt. This lion-identification was making me more and more upset. I was determined to leave. These phases, moods, and conditions were all the divine *kriyas* of Siddha Yoga, coming from the grace of a Siddha, but because I did not know this I was confused when I should have been happy.

Shortly afterward I saw a *tonga* coming across the fields. I could see the driver sitting in front, but could not make out who the passenger was. The *tonga* came near the mango tree. Somebody got down, and I saw that it was Harigiri Baba, a very strange *avadhuta* and a great Siddha yogi. My mind was filled with joy. I got off the swing and stood there waiting for him. He started to call out to me from the *tonga*, "O King, O Emperor, O Swami, get up, get up," and saying this, he burst into peals of laughter.

This great saint was all-knowing. He was always laughing. He used to wander along river banks, wearing an expensive pair of shoes, a silk turban, a coat, and three or four more coats on top of that. Whenever he felt hungry, he would call out to anyone, "Give me something, give me something to eat," and then he would eat. When he finished, he would wash his hands and leave. He was a saint who was like a wandering spirit. He used to collect small stones from the river. He would look at one stone, then at another, and say, "Yes . . . very good, you are worth two hundred thousand." He talked to himself like this and wandered alone, always walking very quickly. He would go to the river bank at 2:00 in the morning, and come back at sunrise. When he spoke, it was hard to understand what he was saying.

Harigiri Baba came up to me, and I bowed to him. I loved Harigiri Baba very much, and he loved me, too. I said, "Baba, things are going badly for me. I am not in a good state." He said, "I know. Give me two *rupees*, and I'll tell you." I knew the way he liked to make jokes. Whenever he came, and you asked him something, he would demand money. Even now he asked for some. I gave him two *rupees*. He spoke to me in Marathi. "O Emperor, you are in a good condition. Things will be very good for you. You will become a god. You've got a beneficial fever. Through coming into contact with it, many people will be cured of their sickness and suffering. You will meet many people." After he had said this, he left. I went with him for some distance, and then he said, "Go, go. You've got to go to come again. Don't be afraid." And so he departed. The people who were nearby started running around, crying, "Harigiri Baba has come."

I went back and sat on the swing. Remembering my lust of that morning and the way I had turned into a lion, my mental turmoil returned. It got steadily worse, for it is the nature of the mind to become like the thing it constantly thinks about. Whatever the mind dwells on, it becomes identified with and takes on its very nature. I am very fond of this verse:

jo mana nāriki or nihārata tau mana hotahi tāhiku rūpā
jo mana kāhusū krodha karai puni tau mana hai tabahī tadarūpā
jo mana māyahi māya raṭai nita tau mana būḍata māyake kūpā
sundara jo mana brahma vichārata tau tava mana hotahi brahmasvarūpā

> The mind that is absorbed night and day in women takes on
>   the nature of a woman,
> The mind that is always angry burns in the fire of anger,
> The mind that is always thinking of *maya* drowns in the pit
>   of *maya*,
> O Sundar, the mind that is continually resting in Brahman
>   eventually becomes That.

This is what that great devotee of Truth, the poet-saint Sundardas says, and it is perfectly true. These two great illusions, sexual excitement and the lion *kriya*, had completely taken over my mind.

I had lived respectably in Yeola for a long time. I was a self-respecting man. "Why," I thought, "should I let people know? I had better go deep into the jungle where no one knows me." So I decided to leave at once. I got up; then I pressed against my heart the photograph of my beloved Gurudev that I used to worship and said, "Forgive me. What else can I do? You are the giver of everything, but I am unlucky." I bowed to him several times and put the photograph back. I looked at my hut and said, "Dear hut, I don't know when I'll see you again. For a long time you have brought me much happiness. I bow to you." I touched the swing and bowed to it also. I embraced my dear friend, the mango tree, and said, "I have passed many days in your shade. What else can I do? I am helpless. Now I have to leave you and go." I went inside the hut, took off my ochre-colored clothes and rolled them up into a bundle, which I hung high in the mango tree, for I felt I should not do anything to tarnish the *dharma* of *sannyasa*. For a long time after this, I wore only white. I left the door of the hut open. I had on a loincloth, a shawl over my shoulders, and a water bowl in my hand. Without saying a word to anyone, I set out toward the east. After a little way, before my hut was out of sight, I stopped to have a look at it. I bowed to it once more. My mind was filled with pain and remorse. I set off again toward the hills, toward a part of the Sahyadri range, and soon found myself right in the midst of them. I wanted to go a long way away. Afterwards, if my body were to fall down somewhere, it would not matter.

On my journey I passed Daulatabad Fort. Then, heading in the direction of the holy place called Ghrishneshvara, near Ellora, I came upon the village of Nagad. I stood on a peak of the Sahyadris, looking north. Below me, I could make out a large sweet lime and orange orchard, large and small mango orchards, and sugarcane plantations. Hunger was gnawing at me, so I set off for one of the orchards. The owner turned out to be a rich farmer who had studied yoga and had great love for *sadhus* and saints. His name was Dagadu Singh. He came up and asked me who I was. Then he invited me to come to his house, where he had some *khicari* made for me with much love.

As I was looking around outside, my eye fell on a small *sadhana* hut. There had been a yogi doing *sadhana* there before. Dagadu Singh made arrangements for me to stay there. When I sat down inside the hut, my legs immediately folded into the lotus posture, and I started meditating. My beloved red aura came and stood before me, and then I heard a voice from within me, "Open that cupboard and read the book you find there." At first I did not pay any attention, but when I heard the voice a second and a third time, my meditation stopped. I opened my eyes and noticed that there was an old cupboard there and that inside it was a book. I took it out and opened it. It opened at a page describing the very *kriyas* that had been happening to me. When I read it, I was supremely happy; in a moment, all my anguish, confusion and worry disappeared. I now understood that everything that had been happening to me was the result of the full blessing of my Gurudev, Bhagavan Sri Nityananda. It was all a part of the process of Siddha Maha Yoga; it was the way to spiritual realization. Now that my problem had been solved, I was able to eat the *khicari* with great satisfaction, and afterward I slept very well.

I stayed in Nagad for some time, doing my *sadhana*. Now I understood that the onset of sexual desire was connected with the process of becoming an *urdhvareta*, from which one gets the power to give Shaktipat. When the *svadhishthana chakra* is pierced, sexual desire becomes very strong, but this happens so that the flow of sexual fluid may be turned upward and the *sadhaka's* lust destroyed forever. When I realized the importance and significance of this process, I became very happy. What more can I write? The ecstasies I had had before came back to me. The naked woman I had seen in meditation had caused so many difficulties only because of my ignorance and confusion of mind. She was, in fact, Mahadevi, the great Goddess Kundalini. I begged forgiveness of the Mother and recited a hymn in praise of Her. From then on, my meditation became very good.

The next day Mother Kundalini stood in the red aura again, but this time I could see Her supremely divine beauty. She was the lovely power of divine grace. As I gazed at Her, I realized my good fortune and bowed to Her, whereupon She merged into the red light. Now this Shakti became my Guru. It was only because my heart was naked, lacking true knowledge, that She had appeared naked to me. The feeling of lust had arisen in me because I had not realized that She was the great Shakti Kundalini. I had taken Her for a mortal, an ordinary woman of the world, and my agony was a result of that ignorance. But now that was all over.

Nagad was a solitary and beautiful place. My meditation progressed automatically. I studied books such as *Mahayoga Vijnana*, containing descriptions of some experiences which are helpful for the yoga of meditation. I sent for other, similar books, such as *Yogavani* and *Shaktipat*. Mahayoga has a very important place in Shaivite philosophy. In the *Shivasutras*, *Pratyabhijnahridayam*, *Tantraloka*, *Shivadrishti*, and other works, one can read what the saints say, in the light of their own experiences, about Shaktipat, the grace of a Siddha, and the dynamic play of Mother Kundalini.

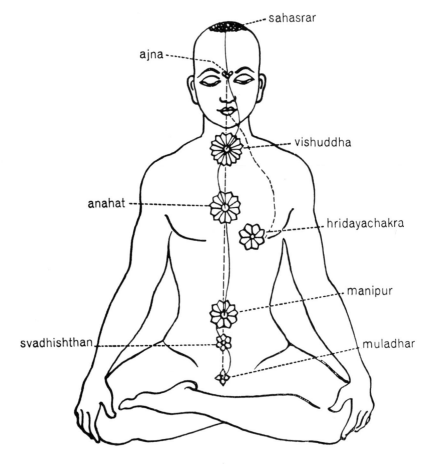

Subtle Centres of Consciousness

Six

Spontaneous Yogic Movements

Now my practice of yoga started to progress very quickly. Three things
had combined to bring this about: divine Shaktipat, the grace of a
great Siddha, and a burning desire to attain God. Before I had lacked
one thing: knowledge about the experiences and the yogic *kriyas* that
happen after Shaktipat. Now that I had read the books that explained
it all to me, what was there to hold me back? My *sadhana* advanced
with the speed of a great river in flood. I had new *kriyas* every day.

I got up every morning at 3:00 to sit for meditation, and as soon
as I sat down, I was seized by a powerful force. As this force overtook
me, the red aura shone. In the middle of the red aura, an oval white
shape that I had not seen before, would appear and disappear, appear
and disappear. After that, there would be just the red aura again. I
would worship my Guru with great joy, and as I worshiped him within
and without, all the fluctuations of my mind would cease. After this,
the three *bandhas* came automatically. My heel locked itself against
my anus, forcing it to contract. By this *kriya*, which is called the
mula bandha, the *apana* is drawn upward. It equalizes the upward-
flowing movement of the *prana* with the downward-flowing movement
of *apana,* and through this destroys old age and sickness. When a
sadhaka sits in the lotus posture and masters the *prana* through this
position, he acquires the capacity to stabilize himself in the state of
thoughtlessness. The frog movement also occurs in this position.

Simultaneously with this, my breath was expelled and my stomach drawn in, so that a small pit was formed. It felt as if air were being drawn up from the region below my navel. This *kriya* is called the *uddiyana bandha* and is given much importance in the Hatha Yogic texts. It is even said in these texts that one can conquer death by it. It purifies the *prana* and the *nadis*. When the *nadis* are purified, the gastric fire begins to blaze, and when the *prana* is purified, the mind stops wandering and becomes stable. After the *uddiyana bandha*, my chin was pressed down hard on my throat. This *kriya* is called the *jalandhara bandha*. It too is very important. Normally, the drops of nectar that trickle down from the *sahasrara* are consumed by the fire of the sun in the navel *chakra*, but this *bandha* seals off its passage, so that the fire can no longer burn the nectar to ashes. With its help, the yogi's mind soon becomes unconscious, which means it attains stillness. These three *bandhas—mula, uddiyana* and *jalandhara—*are very beneficial.

Gradually my *prana* and *apana* became balanced. I also gained complete mastery of the lotus posture. It is said that only when a yogi can hold this posture for three hours has he really mastered it. In the three *bandhas*, I hopped like a frog around my hut with my legs fixed in the lotus posture. By this time, every *kriya* that came made me very happy. I also experienced a variety of *mudras* in my meditation—*maha mudra, maha bandha, mahavedha, viparitakarani mudra, vajroli mudra*. On some occasions I would press one heel against my anus and, stretching out the other leg, grasp my foot with both hands, my head between my arms. This was the *maha mudra*, which forces the Kundalini into the *sushumna* along with the *prana*. Through the *maha mudra*, all the *nadis* are activated and physical inertia dispelled. It aids the retention of semen. The body becomes calm and glowing, the digestive fire gets stronger, the senses become easier to control, and the process of aging is slowed down. When practiced constantly, it eradicates diseases such as tuberculosis, leprosy, piles, hernia, dyspepsia, and spleen trouble. On other occasions I would fold one leg and put the foot on the opposite thigh, at the same time filling my abdomen with air. My chin would lock in *jalandhara bandha*, and my breath would be held, then slowly released. This is called the *maha bandha mudra*. It sends the *prana* into the *sushumna*, makes the body strong and the bones firm. I would also do the *maha-vedha bandha*, which is the *uddiyana bandha* practiced during the *maha bandha*. After exhaling all the air from my lungs, the breath was held outside in the external *kumbhaka*. Through this *bandha*, too, the *prana* goes into the central nerve, and the central nerve and all the three knots —Brahma, Vishnu, and Rudra—are pierced. The Kundalini then travels up to the *sahasrara* and back again. This *bandha* gives mastery over *prana* and arrests old age. Sometimes I would put my hands on the ground, palms upward, put my head on them, and raise both legs straight up. I would remain steady for some time in this position. It is called the *viparitakarani mudra* or *shirshasana*. It brings many benefits. It makes the digestive fire fiercer and prevents wrinkles and grey hair. It stops the nectar of the *sahasrara* from flowing downward, and destroys old age. Sometimes from this position my palms would be placed against the ground and I would push myself up on my arms, my head hanging down between them. This is known as the *vajroli mudra*, which gives sure control over the semen and prevents it from flowing downward by developing the power to retain it. It gives long life to the *sadhaka*.

I also experienced a number of different breathing movements, some of which I will describe. There was one, called the *bhujangini mudra*, in which I would open my mouth wide and drink in air. There was the *nabho mudra*, in which my tongue was stuck against my palate and my breath retained. This exercise destroys disease and enables the tongue to enter the nasal pharynx; it is the first step toward the *khechari mudra*. At times I would roll my tongue into the shape of a crow's bill and suck air inwards. This is known as *kaki* or *sheetali mudra*, which prolongs life, purifies the blood, prevents the formation of cysts, and eliminates fever and bile disorders. Occasionally my forehead would throb terribly, and my eyes would roll up and focus on the spot between the eyebrows. This is the *shambhavi mudra*. It brings great comfort and makes the mind steady; through it a yogi becomes like Shambhu, or Shiva. As the mind concentrates on the space between the eyebrows, one attains the state of *atma chaitanya*, or consciousness of the Self.

My identification with a lion had become stronger still. I roared so much that the cows nearby broke their ropes and ran helter-skelter,

dogs barked madly, and people rushed to my hut. They were astonished to find that it was only Babaji roaring so loudly. I didn't care
whether I gave *darshan* or not, for I was having constant *darshan* of
the mighty processes of Kundalini. I meditated three times a day; at
3:00 in the morning, at 11:00, and then from 7:00 to 9:00 at night.
Sometimes I would zigzag along the ground like a snake, sometimes
hop like a frog, sometimes roar like a tiger. My mind was held spellbound watching the extraordinary inner moods of Goddess Chiti.

I also saw the red aura during these meditations and, more and
more often, the oval white light, which was extremely beautiful. Gradually this light became steadier. I began to experience an unusual kind
of sleep in meditation. My dear Guru, Mother Kundalini Shakti, of
whom I had been so afraid when I had seen Her as a naked woman,
would sometimes appear, and I would remain absorbed in my meditation. Because I did not feel satisfied without knowing more about
meditative states, I asked for many different books.

I went to see another great saint I knew, named Zipruanna. He
was a great Siddha. He used to go naked and spent his time meander-
ing through the lanes of Nasirabad village. He was revered by everyone as a great being and addressed as "Anna" by young and old alike.
He used to live where there were no people, in dilapidated houses and
huts away from the villagers. He had attained a very high state of
yoga. He was farsighted, which is to say he knew about past and future
events. His body had been burned so pure by the fire of yoga that no
filth would touch it. He had raised his body to such a high state that
I marveled at him; the inner Self of yogis is free from stain, and even
Zipruanna's body had this stainless purity. The first time I visited him,
he was defecating in a corner; as I approached, he began to rub his
faeces all over his body. I sat down quite close to him and found that
he emitted a sweet fragrance—he didn't smell bad at all. The next time
I went to see him, he was sitting on a rubbish dump. Even then the
filth would not touch him. I didn't have the courage to go up close; so
I stood at a distance. After a little while, he came down off the rubbish
heap. I washed his feet. A fragrance like the *ashtagandha* (a fragrant
herb) was coming from his body. Zipruanna had great love for me.
Even now I still wonder at the attainments of that great soul. I once
asked him, "Anna, why are you sitting in that filth?" He replied,

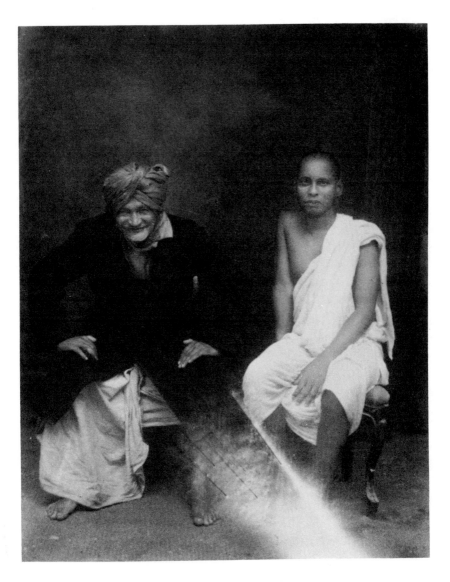

Swami Muktananda with Hari Giri Baba

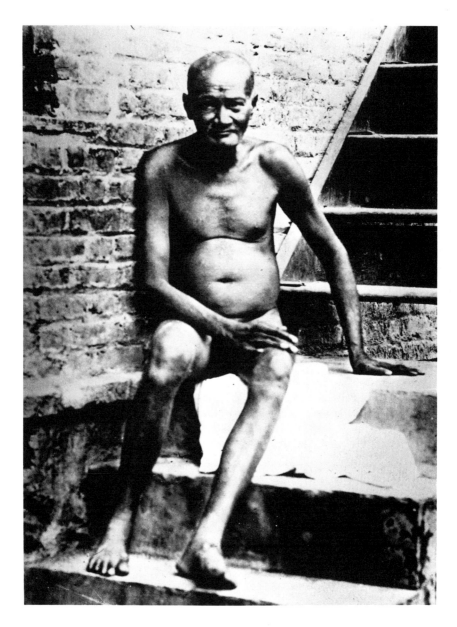

Zipruanna

"Muktananda, the filth that's inside is far worse than this. Think about it. Man's body is just a bag of shit and piss. Isn't it?" I fell silent. Zipruanna was a great *avadhuta*, the crown jewel among saints.

Now, I went to see him again. He greeted me very affectionately, pressing his body to mine. I told him all my experiences in the hut at Suki. He said, "This is the blessing, the initiation, the grace or Shaktipat of a great saint. When you receive such a great blessing, these processes occur. It is normal to see a great conflagration, ghosts, demons, *yakshas*, cobras, *kinnaras*, and all the phantoms of Shiva's army, and this has happened to you." When I asked him about my trouble with lust, he answered, "Only with rare aspirants does the generative organ erect itself and dig into the navel. It is due to the extraordinary divine grace of yoga. Don't underestimate the generative organ. It is the organ that generates all beings and determines whether you are a man or a woman. Without it, a man is a useless eunuch. A man should respect his generative organ; he should restrain and control it as much as possible. When it digs into the navel and remains there for a length of time, all the seminal fluid in the testicles starts to flow upward toward the heart. It is heated in the gastric fire and passes right up to the brain, where it strengthens the sensory nerves. By its strength, the yogi's memory and intelligence are increased." Then he went on, "O Swami, such a man is called an *urdhvareta*. You will become a Guru in the future and will be able to bless others through this power. As a result of the process called *vajroli*, which has happened to you, you will be able to store up the inner Shakti and give the Shaktipat initiation. All your agonies of lust were in fact the great Shakti Kundalini expelling your previous sexual appetites from you. Now, instead of lust, love will surge within you. And from the rays of your love, many others will feel love."

I told him about the naked woman appearing in meditation. I explained that before meditation I had put on the armor of Shiva and closed off all the different directions. How then had the naked woman come through? As I asked this, Baba Zipruanna made a humming sound and he lit up. In a grave voice he answered, "Swami, no one can enter the radiant city of your meditation. No one can go into the luminous land of Goddess Chiti Shakti except Chiti Herself, the deity who is filled with Chiti, and the Guru. It was your own understanding about the nature of woman that confused you. Why do you worry about whether a woman is naked or clothed? The Goddess takes on all forms. When you saw that woman, you should have remembered Goddess Chiti Shakti and looked at Her. No one can gain entry there. It is your attitude that bears fruit according to your conviction. From now on, you should understand whatever forms you see, good or bad, to be forms of Chiti. If you see this naked woman in your heart as the supreme Goddess, then She will show Her divine form. Chiti Shakti can perform innumerable miracles. You must have seen how fast those tiny, fine, subtler than subtle red particles move inside you. Later, you will see countless different worlds in Her. She is the power of Consciousness, who assumes endless forms in a second and who shows all shapes in the One; She is the supreme *maya*, the mother of yoga, Kundalini. O Swami, whatever happened to you was good; everything that will happen in the future will be good. Always remember the real form and nature of the Kundalini.

"Listen to another thing. A yogi on the path of the Siddhas should always remember that anything he sees in the light of the inner heart through the inspiration of Chiti is Chiti in Her fullness. It may be high or low, good or bad, acceptable or repulsive, beautiful or ugly, beneficial or harmful, but it is all Chiti. Nothing can be formed without Chiti. All forms and movements that take place there, whatever they may mean to you, are nothing but the Goddess Chiti."

When I heard this great wisdom from "Zipreshvara," Lord Zipru, I fell at his feet. How wise, how true they were! What an insight into reality he had given me! "Oh my Baba," I cried, embracing him. He sat me down on his lap, licked my head, and passed his hand over it. "Your glory will reach the heavens," he said. In those days, I used to get very bad headaches, but from then on I never had them again.

Zipruanna had solved all my problems for me. I had great faith in him and great reverence for him. I loved him like my Guru. It was he who had sent me to Bhagavan Nityananda. "Everything that you have to do will be fulfilled with him," he had said. "You have a glorious and shining future there."

My dear students of Siddha Yoga, listen carefully. Once you have received the grace of a Guru, you have nothing to fear. You just have to remember one thing—in Siddha Yoga you should obey your Guru. This is a basic principle that you should keep in your mind always. Remember what Anna asked me, "How can such a large woman enter the subtle region of the inner heart? How can an ordinary woman pierce your armor, forged of mantra and *tantra*, which guards all directions?" In the red light that comes with the awakening of Chiti Kundalini, you will see everything. Can you see it if Chiti does not want you to? Think and remember. The space within the heart is extremely subtle, and only the Kundalini can enter there. You should think of everything you see, everything you undergo, and all the *kriyas* that come to you as the blessings of the divine Goddess Chiti, and offer them up to Her. Know that everything which happens to you is entirely for your own good. Mentally, you should bow in reverence to all the forms Chiti assumes, to all the *kriyas* She causes, to the shapes, colors, and states She reveals, understanding them all as manifestations of Herself. If you do this, you will soon become calm and peaceful; if you think they are different from Chiti, you will suffer the remorse that Muktananda did.

After my visit to Zipruanna, I returned to my beloved hut at Nagad and took up my *sadhana* with great confidence. I began to have very good meditations. The oval white shape the size of a thumb would appear and remain for a long time, surrounded by the red aura the size of my body. I enjoyed meditation more and more. Everything I saw I took as the divine Chiti and mentally bowed to Her.

My happiness kept growing. Sometimes I wanted to dance. Why this desire came I do not know, but it filled my whole body. While I was feeling this, I would see the red aura and the thumb-sized white flame as well. Many physical *kriyas, mudras,* and Hatha Yoga *asanas* occurred in the physical body. I did *asanas* every two or three days rather than every day.

In the red aura, I later saw the tremendous radiance of the golden inner *akasha* and the shimmering brightness of the silver *akasha*. I saw places in the Himalayas that I had never visited and peaks I had never seen. I was acquiring a new inner eye, and although I did not know exactly what it was, with this new eye I could see many places within the red aura. In an individual, this red aura is three and a half arm-lengths long, but on the universal scale it extends from east to west, north to south, above and below, and contains the whole body of the cosmos.

In meditation, I saw some of the holy places of India. I had now reached a new stage in meditation, and along with the red and white lights, I saw many vast lands with mountain ranges covered with jungles and woods. I was, in other words, having visions in meditation and was quite conscious of all that was happening. I was also very happy.

My body got gradually thinner, but as it became purer, it also became stronger. Sometimes I would get a slight fever or cold, but it would not last for long. I would also get attacks of dysentery, but they too would clear up quickly. All the ailments I got at that time were cured by meditation.

I now understood that it is the gross body, the description of which we may read in Vedanta, which is seen in meditation as that red aura. All *kriyas* happen in this body. The *jiva*, or individual soul, in this body is represented by "A," the first letter of *Aum*, and its name is *vishva*. This is the body of the waking state, and is the instrument of gross experiences and actions. An ignorant man identifies himself with this body. Because he doesn't know the inner Self, the Witness-consciousness, he thinks, "I am my body." Yet, he who knows a pitcher as "this pitcher" is different from the pitcher; likewise, he who perceives a car as "this car" is different from it, even if he is sitting inside it. In exactly the same way, the One who lives inside the red light, who is the Witness of it, who knows it as "this," is different from it. He is the pure divine principle, the Godhead, which is the goal of meditation. Actually, the distinction between spirit and matter has meaning only until true knowledge is attained. After that, one understands that both the seer and the seen are the one supreme Consciousness, Parashakti, the witnessing Being, who by occupying the gross body appears to be gross but is in fact the Self of all, whom the scriptures describe as *vijñānamānandaṁ brahma*—"the Absolute, possessing knowledge and bliss."

The Kundalini Shakti, which is awakened by the Guru's grace, performs new tasks every day. She enters the system of the 72,000 *nadis*, purifies and strengthens the *nadis* that carry blood and *prana*, and transmits vital energy into them. In this way She purifies the body.

She enters the *sushumna* within the spinal column and, piercing the *chakras* through Her own force, changes the whole condition of the body and makes it fit for the spiritual path. Practitioners of the Siddha Science should remember that She will put everything right in one's ordinary life as well. She takes care of one's children and helps one acquire all the necessities of life. She gives the understanding needed to deal with any situation with which one is faced. Scriptural texts have distinguished the worldly from the spiritual, but when one has complete understanding, these two become one. This external world is the play of Chiti, filled with Chiti; it is not different from Chiti, and it is the manifestation of Chiti. Chiti is constantly assuming ever-new forms through the unending stretch of beginningless time. The universe is the very body of Chiti. Siddha students should remember that concepts such as "matter," "the void," "perishable," or "the seen" exist only in the absence of perfect knowledge.

Revered Tukaram Maharaj said, "I meditated, and through the experience given me by this inner Shakti, I realized that everything is God Himself." He wrote in one of his verses:

> *rakta śveta kṛṣṇa pīta prabhā bhinna*
> *chinmaya añjana sudalem ḍorām*
> *teṇem añjanaguṇem divyadṛṣṭi jhālī*
> *kalpanā nivālī dvaitādvaita*
> *deśakālavastubheda māvaralā*
> *ātmā nirvāralā viśvākāra*
> *na jhālā prapañcha āhe parabrahma*
> *ahamsoham brahma ākaralem*
> *tattvamasi vidyā brahmānanda sānga*
> *tenchi jhālā ange tukā ātām*

It means: "When by the grace of my Guru, Sri Babaji, I saw the extremely subtle, Consciousness-filled divine light of the Self, which is different from the red, white, black, and yellow lights, the lotion of pure Consciousness bathed my eyes. Then my vision became divine, and the imaginary distinction between unity and duality vanished. My sense of difference regarding space, time, and substance totally disappeared. There is no space, no time, no substance; there is no diversity. My Self appeared as the universe, and the universe, which we call objective reality, appeared as my Self. There is no outer world. Only the Absolute exists. I had the direct experience of 'I am He, I am Brahman.' I, Tukaram, became Brahmananda, the transcendental bliss that is attained through the understanding of the Vedantic declaration, 'Thou art That.'

The world, which during *sadhana* appears differentiated, becomes God when one reaches full realization. Tukaram says, 'I am perfect in my own being.'"

We, too, should penetrate in meditation the thumb-sized white light within the red aura and win that perfect experience so that we may see God pervading the whole world as the world.

Through the *sadhana* of Chiti our world becomes good. This is no exaggeration. Sri Shankaracharya says:

> sarvo'pi vyavahārastu brahmaṇā kriyate janaiḥ
> ajñānānna vijānanti mṛudeva hi ghaṭādikam
>
> *(Aparokshanubhuti, 65)*

All the activities of men are possible only because of the existence of God, but because of their ignorance they are not aware of it. A pot or any other earthen vessel is simply earth.

It is like a spider who produces a web from inside itself, lives in it, and finally draws it back into itself.

Since the whole world is filled with Chiti, since all parts of the physical world are Chiti Herself, since Chiti appears as all the men and women in the world, it follows that, when She is awakened within you, your life will naturally be prosperous and happy. This is not an exaggeration; it is the simple truth. When you become worthy of Parashakti's grace, then in your journey through life, in your work and in your pleasures, with wife or husband, you can create a world that is happy and full of bliss.

Day by day, my meditation increased in length, and each day there were new experiences. Somewhere within the red aura I found a divine eye and could see the whole universe before me. While I was in Nagad, sitting in meditation, I could see my hut in Suki. My meditation was so extensive that the whole universe seemed to be only a small portion of it. *Sadhakas*, don't doubt me, don't wonder at me. Let me give you an example from modern technology, which is well-known to you, which you utilize and consider to be reliable. On a small radio you can listen to a broadcast from Bombay, even when you are a long way away. You turn the knob a fraction, and you are listening to Delhi. You turn it a little bit more, and you get Calcutta. You are completely aware of this. If you change the wave-band, you can listen to news from England and America. All you have to do to get broadcasts from different cities or countries is to turn the knob an inch. If by sitting at home and using a piece of material equipment you are able to listen to broadcasts from all over the world, what is there to stop you listening to the news of different places through meditation? And now we have a new device—television. This is a further confirmation. On television you can see the newsman and the place where he is speaking from. So if you can see the world within the inner light in meditation, there's nothing extraordinary about it.

As I meditated, I went into a new *tandra* state. I began to see a yellow light. Sometimes I would see the red and white lights mixed. As I contemplated the yellow light, which was very beautiful, I saw more, different lands. This new condition was like *samadhi*, but I was fully conscious and still distinguishing between the perceiver and the perceived. After having been in this state for a while, I would feel great joy. It banished all my fatigue. I began to increase the length of my meditation still more. My body was getting thinner, and even my calves were losing flesh. The seven bodily elements were being purified. I was eating the same amount of food, but excreting less. My faeces were as hard as wood and no longer smelled very much. My sweat was also less pungent. Even though my body looked just as robust, it felt lighter and more energetic. Throwing away all my cares in the drunkenness of love, I would sometimes dance wildly in the solitude of the orchard.

I had mastered the lotus posture and was able to sit in it for three hours. Then my tongue began to undergo a new and strange *kriya*. Sometimes it reached down to my heart, and at other times it was held up against the palate, but after meditation it would return to its usual place. Many strange *kriyas* like this took place. In the *tandra* state I saw more visions. My faith in my Gurudev and surrender to Chiti were growing, and I was developing new energy and courage in *sadhana*. In meditation a shape appeared to me and told me, "When your tongue moves downward, it is performing the holy yogic task of opening the heart lotus, and when it goes up into the nasal pharynx, that is the *khechari mudra*. This process will bring you to a high state." When the tongue is held upward, the way to the *sahasrara* is opened. This is the way by which the awakened Kundalini goes to meet the supreme Lord, Parashiva, who is enthroned in the midst of a thousand rays in the *sahasrara*. Sometimes I saw the deities and lights of all the *chakras*. These *kriyas* were not dependent on my will, but were gifts of the Guru's grace, inspired by supreme Shakti. Sometimes during meditation my legs would feel stiff and dead, but afterward they returned to normal.

One thing I always did was to sit in the meditation posture for the full period, even if I couldn't meditate or if my mind was unable to concentrate itself. I benefited a lot from this. My dear Siddha students, remember that when you sit in the lotus posture for three hours, the 72,000 *nadis* are completely purified.

The purification of the *nadis* is the greatest of all purifications. There can be no lasting happiness while the *nadis* are still impure, while they are filled with diseased, foul-smelling, unwholesome filth. I will give you an analogy. Can you feel peaceful and at ease if in every room and corner of your house there is a horrible smell, if it is buzzing with mosquitoes and insects and pervaded by the stink of drains or toilets? It is the same with your body. If it is filthy and prone to all kinds of ailments, if you are permanently sniffling with a cold and your nose needs three or four handkerchiefs every hour to keep it clean, if there is the rank smell of unevacuated waste coming from your entrails to sicken your neighbors, can there be any happiness in such a body? Can you remove that inner stench with scents and perfumes? Can you make your face bright and attractive by rubbing on creams and powders and lipsticks like actors and actresses? Remember: *sarīramādyaṁ khalu dharmasādhanam*—"It is the body which is the principle means for *dharma*."

When the *nadis* are purified, the *prana* is automatically purified. Then *pranayama* naturally follows. In the *sadhana* of Shaktipat, through the Guru's grace, *pranayama* comes automatically during meditation. After the *nadis* and the *prana* have been purified, the tendencies of the four psychic instruments also become pure. Then the level of meditation goes higher and higher. For this reason you should devote a lot of time to the mastery of the meditation posture.

Next, I started to feel a kind of warmth growing in my body. It grew so hot that it started to burn me everywhere. No matter what method I tried to cool my body, it went on burning as if on fire. I became very thin. Phlegm began to run from my mouth. I took rice-water instead of solid food. My body was getting so hot from this burning Shakti that I didn't get any relief even when I sat in a pool of cold water. At that point I received a message from Bhagavan Nity-ananda in Ganeshpuri. The people of Yeola had been astonished by the way I had gone away, telling no one and leaving my hut with the door open. They had told Nityananda Babaji about this and also that I was, at the moment, in the neighborhood of Chalisgaon. His message said that my *sadhana* was going well, that all my experiences were authentic, and that I should pursue my *sadhana* with great courage. It made me very happy. Later I got another loving message from dear Gurudev, brought by Sri Narayan Sendo, one of his greatest devotees, of whom I was very fond. He took a bottle of genuine *khus* scent from his pocket and gave it to me. "Why have you brought this?" I asked him, and he answered, "Swami, I got it for Bhagavan Nity-ananda, but when I gave it to him, he said, 'Go to Chalisgaon and Nagad and give it to him,' so please take it." I took it, feeling it was a gift of grace from Bhagavan. I opened it and rubbed on a little of it. It was of a very good quality. I dabbed it all over myself, and a won-derful fragrance filled the air. We talked about Bhagavan Nityananda, and I heard all the news about him. After this, my meditation became more intense. The next day, when I was meditating and in the *tandra* state, Bhagavan came to me. He handed me the same bottle of *khus* scent and said, "Your meditation will release more heat. It is the burning radiance of yoga. Use some scent every day." I was very pleased to get the scent and this advice in meditation like that.

Every day after meditation I would eat and then sit under a mango tree and read a book about yoga. I came across a recommendation that yogis should wear sweet-smelling flowers, because they and their scent alleviate the heat generated in yoga. This made me think about the customs of our culture. This was the reason why flowers are placed on the Lord in the Indian ritual of worship. It also explains why devotees take expensive, fragrant flowers when they go for the *darshan* of a saint. I also understood why sandalwood paste is applied to the feet. So from then on I always put on a garland of *mogra* flowers when I sat to meditate in the morning, and after meditation I would put on either *khus* or *heena* scent.

My meditation got much better. I saw a mixed yellow and blue light and passed into a wonderful *tandra* state. The happiness of *tandra* is far greater than any happiness you can find in eating or drinking or in fulfilling any desire in the waking state and far greater than the state of sleep, which gives you dreams at night. It is the happiness of the state of *tandra*-meditation. Sometimes I would see the state of sleep clearly, and I saw that its pleasure was nothing next to the pleasure of the sleeplike state of *tandra* and that all its happiness was unreal. Then I began to experience the delight of Tandraloka more and more.

Sometimes I would see a beautiful, slender, silver-colored tube, standing like a pillar from the *muladhara* to the throat. It was very fascinating, and I wondered how such a slender tube could be permeated with the silvery light. Sometimes I would see a god in each *chakra*, and feel a slight pain there. Sometimes I would look right into my body at the nervous, circulatory, excretory, and digestive systems. The same multi-colored light spread throughout all the *nadis* and illuminated them, so that I could see them. I could also see the Shakti vibrating in them with increasing intensity.

Everyday, meditation would begin with currents of *prana* spreading through my body, and then I would see the red and white lights. I started to see still more worlds in meditation and would often see *Shivalingas* and other deities. When the white light dawned, my meditation would go into the subtle body, and I would see the subtle form of the outer phenomenal world within me. Then, in this state, I would go right into *tandra*, where I would see strange cobras and terrifying snakes of all kinds, and these would frighten me.

After meditation I always went carefully over my experiences. I talked much less because I spent so much time reading, meditating, and resting. Whenever a group of devotees came, I would talk with them, and this meant that I did not meditate at regular times. As a result, the *tandra* state would not come, and there would be less delight in meditation. (Readers should note that from now on I will describe the place of the *tandra* state as Tandraloka, the world of *tandra*.) If I was disturbed by some problem of the mind or of the outside world, I was unable to meditate or visit Tandraloka and I would feel dejected as a result. So I stopped seeing people and getting into conversations.

In meditation I was sometimes able to see events in the outer world, and I began to understand this world much better. I saw the lotus of the heart in the middle of the white flame. The most fleeting glimpse of that divine and radiant light was enough to hold me spellbound, and on the occasions when it went on sparkling with its lightning speed, I would be overcome with bliss and rapture. If I happened to be sitting near a mango tree when this happened, I would lovingly embrace it.

Gradually my meditation left the gross body and entered the subtle body; it left Rakteshwari, the goddess of the red aura, for Shveteshwari, the goddess of the white flame, and this thumb-sized white flame was always before me. The subtle body, which is shaped like a thumb and which I have hitherto spoken of as Shveteshwari, is the means by which the individual soul experiences the dream state and enjoys some rest after the labor of its waking hours. It is the subtle body spoken of in Vedanta, and it supports the gross, or physical, body. It is represented by "*u*," the second letter of *Aum*. The individual soul in this body is called *taijasa*. Its seat is in the throat, and the white flame may be seen there in a vision or in a dream. Without the experience of this white flame, Vedanta is a lame and second-hand philosophy: *darvī pākarasaṁ yathā*—"It is like a ladle that does not know the taste of the food it serves."

My meditation on the subtle plane gradually deepened. To begin with, I slept a bit too much in meditation, but this soon passed. I began to have visions of future happenings—a fire breaking out somewhere, or a motor accident. A day or two after I had seen such things, I would hear about them as events that had happened. It made me enjoy meditation still more; I was filled with praise for the wonders of meditation.

One day as I began to meditate, I saw a beautiful baby boy swinging in a cradle. He was a small baby about a year and a half old, and he wore a pearl necklace and a golden crown. I had never seen anyone so beautifully adorned. His cradle was also of gold and was studded with the nine jewels. There was nobody else with him. I saw the enchanting child surrounded by lights of many colors. I can still remember him. He was turned toward me, laughing ecstatically and beckoning me with his tiny eyes. How joyful this meditation was! That day, I went beyond Tandraloka and saw nothing for a long time—only a pure untainted state. My meditation ended. I closed my eyes again and tried to visualize the baby with my mind's eye, but I couldn't. I was convinced that the baby was Sri Hari. After seeing him, my *sadhana* got even better, especially for the two or three days that followed. On one occasion I saw heaped up strings of pearls; on another, I saw a wonderfully beautiful cow suckling a calf the same color as the baby in the golden cradle.

Now I began to feel very curious beforehand about what I was going to see in meditation. During the day I would say to myself, "Why doesn't evening come soon so I can meditate?" and then at night I would think, "Why doesn't morning come soon so I can meditate?" Some of the things I saw were so captivating that I began to be addicted to meditation. Afterward I would go over my visions again and again. My body would thrill with excitement, and I would rapturously congratulate myself on my good fortune. Thus most of my days and nights were spent in meditation and in recollection of my visions.

Eight

Krishneshwari: The Black Light

My white meditation was followed by a black meditation. Here, "krishna" does not refer to Lord Sri Krishna but to the *krishna* (black) color of the light. A black light the size of a fingertip appeared, which marked the next stage in meditation. My mind would spontaneously focus on my heart, or on the space between the eyebrows. First, my attention would be fixed on the red, white, and black lights. I would see the white flame within the red aura, and the black light within the white flame. Sometimes while I was looking at these, I would also see many lights of different colors, but my meditation would become truly stable only when I concentrated on the black light. I felt peaceful, but at the same time I was so eager to know what I was going to see next that my mind was not as quiet as it might have been. During this period I would see in meditation a deep and terrifying darkness such as I had never seen in the outside world. This darkness made me frightened of meditating, but even so, I would remain in it for long periods at a time. Then suddenly the scene would change and the familiar red, white, and black lights would come. I rejoiced in their radiance again and again. During all this I began to feel a strong pain between the eyebrows, and for several days the *chakras* situated there and in the head continued to ache. I don't know why my eyes rolled around continuously, causing me great pain. Both eyes would roll upward and the pupils would spin like wheels. Then there came a new experience; when my eyes spun I would feel the *prana* moving gently between my throat and the space between my eyebrows. I smelled many different sweet odors; I don't know whether or not they can be found in this world of ours. Sometimes other people would smell a fragrance floating around me, and my meditation hut became permeated with fragrance. Every now and then my eyes would stop spinning and roll upward so that I could see inside my skull. I saw a dazzlingly bright sun as well as some stars. Then my meditation would stop. I would compose myself, walk outside my hut, and sit under the mango tree, where I would reflect upon the things I had seen, both great and small.

One morning as my mind was fixed on the black goddess within the red and white lights, I saw a city surrounded by impenetrable darkness. I do not know how far inside I went, but I covered a considerable distance. At the end, the scene in the black light suddenly changed. The three lights reappeared together, and as I gazed at them, I found myself in a thick jungle. I was sitting under a tree when a black cobra swiftly slid up to me and bit me. The poison spread through my body, and I could feel that my end was near. Just then, a devotee from Yeola arrived who used to prepare my bath and sometimes cooked my food. He prayed to Parashiva for me, and after his prayer I recovered from this critical state of poisoning. All this was like a scene in a drama, and I can still remember it. Later on I found a book about *sadhana* from which I learned that a snake bite during meditation is a great sign of fearlessness on the path of Siddha Yoga and an important vision. It indicates that the aspirant will steadily advance in meditation.

By now I was sometimes meditating on the white light and sometimes on the black. I saw the mountains around Shree Shailam within the black light, and their large caves inhabited by sages. Sometimes I would see a variety of different lights within the caves of Mount Girnar. Wherever I looked, I saw a beautiful light of mixed blue, red, and yellow, and everything I saw was in the brightness of this divine radiance. Three or four days after I was bitten by the snake, I saw Nagaloka, the world of cobras. There were flower gardens everywhere, full of cobras, and these snakes were all a lustrous blue. I saw one enormous cobra whose color was extremely radiant. Many visions, many cities, appeared like this, bringing me great joy.

When my meditation stopped, I would remain quiet and peaceful, and with the passing of the days, my mind became increasingly calm. I began to see the lights in the waking state as well. Whenever I was thinking intensely about my Guru, or deep in identification with him, I would see the three lights while awake and engaged in my daily tasks. The tide of my bliss continued to rise. The red, the white, and the black lights—Rakta, Shveta, Krishneshwari—both in meditation and while I was awake! If I was wandering about the orchard, I saw the lights. Wherever I looked, they would be shining there! I was filled with wonder. There must have been some magic in the bite of that cobra-king. Perhaps it was to push me further along the path of progress that Shiva Nageshwara, the Lord of cobras, had blessed me.

Next my eardrums were afflicted with a pain that was very intense, but lasted only for a short time. My eyes kept rolling. My upper eyelid would remain fixed above my eye, the lower eyelid below, and I would stay like that without blinking for two hours at a time. My eyes would bulge, and the people who saw me during this period would remark among themselves that I looked angry. I don't know why I looked at everyone with such staring eyes. When I was normal again, people said that I looked gentle. All I could say was that I was neither angry nor gentle.

Events went on in this way—on the one hand, things happening in the *nadis* throughout my body; on the other hand, experiences in meditation, and my relentless pursuit of *sadhana.*

Next I started to visit Chandraloka in meditation. It is quite true that there is a world on the moon. The people living in it are all the same age. I saw many men and women walking along paths covered with flowers in a garden there. They were all young and healthy. The whole time I was at the edge of the garden, looking into it. On the moon there was no heat from the sun, but everything was diffused with a soft and gentle light. Looking at the towns there, I observed that there must be neither rain nor hot sun. All the houses were made of gold and silver. I did not see any old people there.

Ten

Vision of Hell and the God of Death

A few days passed in this way, and I felt very happy. Then, again, I started to meditate on the black light. One day I saw a world that was extremely filthy. Siddha students should read this passage carefully. That day, when I sat for meditation, my whole body shook violently, just as if I were possessed by a god or a bad spirit. In that state, I saw in meditation that I was traveling a very long way, but I did not know where I was going or how. Although my physical body was still sitting in meditation, I arrived at a place that was utterly filthy, filled with excreta. I found myself standing in a heap of refuse. I am fully aware of what I am saying. Muktananda says: Siddha students, read this carefully. Wherever I looked I saw nothing but excreta. God knows for how many ages these turds had been piling up there. Just as in Mahableshwar you can see mountains all around from whichever point you are standing, so now I could see piles and piles of excrement all around, as though it had been accumulating there for many years. As I moved a bit, my feet began to sink into it.

A revolting stench was coming from all sides, and this made me want to vomit. I started to feel giddy. The paths were rough and crude, and what water there was, was mixed with excreta. I saw only a few men and women, all of them naked. Some were sitting on heaps of dung, looking sad and ugly. I was filled with loathing at the sight of all this. I stumbled on ahead with great difficulty. There was some light, but the sun was not visible. *Sadhakas*, please remember this experience of mine. When I came to this place, I lost all my radiance. I searched for a way out. With great difficulty, I found one, but that, too, was filled with excreta. Then I saw a hill of dried-out excreta on which men and women were seated. I marveled at all I had seen.

After this, I went to another world where there were woods and gardens filled with fruit and flowers, and many kinds of cows, oxen, horses and other animals. I saw some men there who were about twenty feet tall, dark-skinned, with protruding teeth. They all carried in their hands flashing swords about six feet long and large goads. Some wore silken clothes, some wore animal skins, and others were in ordinary clothes. Their eyes were red with anger. There were no women there, which surprised me a great deal. I also saw some black bull water buffaloes about twenty feet long. Then I saw an extremely fascinating lake, with beautiful chirping birds all around it. Nearby flowed a delightful river. There was a brilliant light everywhere—perhaps the sun's or that of some other star. In the midst of this radiance, I saw a black god sitting on a dark water buffalo decorated with flowers and covered with a silken sheet. The animal's horns were covered with gold and it wore golden anklets on its hoofs. The god wore a red *dhoti*, a sacred thread, and a jeweled crown on his head. He was about ten feet away from me. I smiled when I saw him, and he too smiled at me, raising his hands in the gesture of fearlessness. I was overjoyed and full of gladness, for I had seen Yamaraja, the lord of death. After a little while, two of his attendants came and led me out, taking me back through the hellish mire again. Then my meditation stopped. I stepped out of my hut. My heart felt dry, and I tried to drink some water, but I started to vomit. My heart was filled with disgust. I did not eat for three days. Even now I feel disgusted when I remember it.

Meanwhile, my meditation continued in the same way. While going into meditation I would be seized by a wave of Shakti. My tongue would curl upward, my eyes rolling in the same direction, and I would see the lights revealed outside. My meditation kept progressing, and sometimes I got so deeply absorbed in it that fear of death arose in my mind. I would think, "I am going to die, I am going to

Eleven

The Piercing of the Optical Chakras

Next, the pupils of both my eyes became centered together. I began to see one thing with two eyes. In the scriptures this is called *bindu bheda*. After this had happened, a blue light arose in my eyes. This is the necessary preliminary to the *shambhavi mudra*. When the aspirant experiences the *neelodaya*, the dawning of the blue light, it signifies the dawning of his supreme good fortune. When the process starts, some aspirants fear that they may lose their eyesight. With me, my eyes rolled so violently around and around and up and down that it seemed as if they would fall out. Some people saw it happening and they too were frightened. But I put all my trust in the Goddess, believing that it is not I, but She, the Paramatmashakti, the power of God who is within us, who does everything. And so all my fears vanished.

As the eyes revolve, the optical *chakras* are pierced, which pleases their deity. *Sadhakas* should not forget that each one of our senses has its particular deity. While the *chakras* are still unpurified, the deity carries on its work in the ordinary way, but when the *chakras* are purified they become invested with divine powers. When the optical *chakras* are purified by piercing, their deity bestows divine sight on the aspirant, and he becomes clairvoyant.

Now in meditation I felt bliss and also a growing energy. At the same time, the pain in my eyes, ears, and the space between the eyebrows increased. My meditation would be centered first on the red aura, then on the white flame, and then on the black light. When I sat for meditation, I would have some bodily *kriyas*, then the *prana* would flow forcefully through my *nadis*, and my tongue would curl back into the *khechari mudra*; my meditation would then become perfectly steady. I would feel waves of ecstasy welling up inside me. But even though I was completely carried away, I understood everything that was happening to me, and my understanding has not changed in the least today. It is as it was then. Such understanding is very important. Sometimes I felt that my ability to understand was also new, because I remembered even the tiniest details of my experiences. I remained very attentive and tried to understand this power of intuitive intelligence.

By this time, my sexual desire had gone completely, and this was replaced by a new and increasing love; it grew so much that love for everything flowed out from me. I would think to myself, "Isn't this possessiveness, isn't it infatuation and attachment? I have just come to Nagad, so how could I already be so attached to these mango trees?" But as I thought about it, I realized that my tenderness for the mango trees was a reflection of God's love. God loves all things unconditionally, with a great and impartial love. His love is not like the ordinary love of worldly people. Mundane love is not love; it is business, buying and selling. The butcher lovingly fattens his lamb every day, but is this love? He loves only to make money. The milkmaid lovingly feeds her cows and buffaloes, but is this really love and generosity? She does it only to sell their milk. The farmer loves his fields; he works hard on them and gives them seeds. Is that true love or true giving? All these kinds of love are just buying and selling. How can there be any happiness when there is no true love? Love is unmotivated tenderness of the heart. Human love always has some motive behind it. It is not love; it is only selfishness and self-interest. The only pure love is God's love. His very nature is love, His grace is love, His giving is love, and His taking is love. God looks upon the entire universe with the eye of love, and the world is sustained by this ray of His love. When this state of God arises in the aspirant, he, too, feels love for all creatures. There is no longer any feeling of serving or being served. Love is pure compassion; it takes no account of merit.

In meditation there was another marvel: after I had visited the dark black world, which I described before Nagaloka, I saw a decorated elephant before me. It had seven heads and was adorned with beautiful heavenly cloths and huge necklaces made of gold, pearls, and rubies. All its ornaments flashed in the rays of the early morning sun. I contemplated the elephant for a long time, wondering about it. After my meditation I consulted a *Purana* and learned that it was the elephant Airavata from the world of Indra and that seeing it in a vision was very meritorious.

Meditation once again engulfed me. My enthusiasm grew so much that I wanted to spend all day and all night in meditation. But this was not possible, for one needs the strength to endure the extraordinary force, strain, heat and power involved in meditation. One should do only as much meditation as one is capable of bearing, and one should practice good conduct, celibacy, and self-control, and eat pure food. If you cannot discipline yourself, it will be difficult for you to get the full benefit of meditation, to get the full attainment. A meditator should really understand himself and know his own greatness. He should not indulge in unrestrained behavior, laugh and cry a lot, gossip about useless things, eat carelessly, or do whatever he feels like doing. He should not degrade himself, for if he does, he will also degrade the power of divine grace, which is the fruit of great self-discipline. Then he will not be able to perfect the mantra or achieve clairvoyance, the vision of his chosen deity, and worldly prosperity.

I remember how someone once said to me, "Babaji, I have practiced meditation, but I couldn't find any joy in it." Another man said, "I have had a vision in meditation, but it didn't turn out to be true." One man said, "When I sit for meditation, I get frightened." Another said that his worries and anxieties got worse in meditation. I tell everyone who comes to me with complaints like this that they have not properly followed the rules of meditation. My dear Siddha students! All these obstacles arise because of your disrespect for the great Shakti, which has become active within you. If you don't care where you go, if you make friends with the wrong sort of people, the attainment of full realization is prevented. If this were not so, why should some people attain more and some less when the Guru's Shakti that enters them is one and the same?

My eyeballs had been revolving, and now the pupils were centered and had become as one. The eyeballs rolled up and down. Then, while this was happening, a tiny, extremely brilliant dot shot out of my eyes with the speed of lightning and then went back in again. This is a secret, mysterious, and marvelous process. In an instant the tiny blue dot illuminated everything in every direction. If I were sitting facing east, the whole of the east would be lit up. If I were facing south, the whole of the south would be lit up.

Siddha students, how can I tell you about the greatness and glory of that Blue Pearl! It was animated, and faster than a flash of lightning. When I saw it, I was filled with many emotions. Would Rama or Krishna or my especially adored Parashiva come with it? Who was I to meet after Airavata? I was greedy for visions, but still my mind was happy and full of joy and contentment. My days passed differently from before, for my heart was deeply satisfied with the vision of the Blue Pearl, and it told me that I had been blessed with a gift from the Goddess Kundalini. I began to honor everyone in my heart.

When my eyes stopped rolling, they would stay turned upward. I would keep looking upward, and if I looked down it would hurt. Sometimes my eyes stayed open without blinking. I started to feel a pain between the eyebrows, which was so strong that I could not sleep at night. Then a light came in meditation, like a candle flame without a wick, and stood motionless in the *ajna chakra*, the two-petaled lotus between the eyebrows. It was extremely brilliant and beautiful. As I gazed at it, quite forgetful of myself, my vision became blurred. Next to that light is the path that the awakened Kundalini takes on Her way to the *sahasrara*. This is the pathway of the Siddhas, which does not open without the full grace of a Guru. No matter how great your devotion or your *tapasya*, no matter how much you meditate or how many *kriyas* you experience, this path is very difficult to open without the Guru's grace. There is only one way: *gurukripā hi kevalam gurorājna hi sādhanam*—"The Guru's grace is the only way, the Guru's command is the only method."

This *chakra* was also pierced, and the *pranashakti* began to climb higher. I saw the wickless flame constantly before me and was constantly filled with bliss. The place of the flame is the same place where devout Indian women put *kumkum* every day as a symbol of their fidelity in marriage. They put *kumkum* there in the name of their husbands or just because it is customary, but that place is actually the seat of the Guru, and it is there that the presiding deity of the Guru's seat lives, in the form of the two seed syllables "*ham*" and "*ksham.*" We owe our existence to it. The flame is one form of the supreme Gurudev. When our women put *kumkum* there, they are worshiping the supreme Self. Times have changed now, and some women have forgotten this duty. Everything is becoming the opposite of what it once was.

I kept seeing this divine flame, and as I contemplated it, other forms would appear within it, each form within the previous one: first the red aura, then the white flame, then the black light, and finally the Blue Pearl. As I passed through all these different stages, moving ahead, my joy and ecstasy kept increasing.

I was beginning to experience a new kind of bliss. I had frequent visions, which were absolutely authentic. When I saw the Blue Pearl, the condition of my body and mind, and my way of understanding, began to change. I felt more and more delight in myself, and was filled with pure and noble feelings. I started to tire of all forms of external associations and became addicted only to meditation. I always asked myself, "What shall I see today?" This was the only thing I waited for, the only thing I took interest in, the only thing I enjoyed, and it became my daily action and my daily meditation.

One day I sat down to meditate at the *brahma muhurta*, the last hours of the night, and found myself in front of a funeral pyre in a cremation ground. An unknown woman was seated in it. She was surrounded by flames and was being consumed by them, but she was completely absorbed in meditation. I watched her for a long time, and then my meditation stopped.

By now I yearned for meditation as a greedy man yearns for wealth; I thought about it like a man lusting after a girl. I remembered it like a madman who is obsessed with one thing and goes back to it again and again. The next day I decided that henceforth my meditation should start at midnight. My meditation had become so subtle that I could not bear a noise or any kind of disturbance from the outside world. Even if someone spoke softly I was disturbed. If someone laughed or a dog barked, my meditation was interrupted. I felt even the presence of my usual companions as an obstacle and was always thinking what a relief it would be when they went. And so I started to meditate from midnight onward in my hut at Nagad.

I did not meditate out of fear, but with enthusiasm and faith and love. I did not meditate to please anyone or to get any benefits from anyone or to satisfy a desire, sensual or otherwise. I did not meditate to rid myself of any illness, physical or mental, nor to gain fame through the miraculous and supernatural powers I might acquire. No one forced me to meditate. I did not meditate because religion says that it is good to meditate. I meditated solely for the love of God, because I was irresistibly drawn toward the Goddess Chiti Shakti, and to explore my own true nature.

As soon as I sat, I passed into meditation. The presiding deity of each sense organ would come and stand before me. I would see a very special kind of light made up of many colors flashing through the 72,000 *nadis* like lightning. Then would come the red, white, and black lights, and, for a second, the Blue Light. These lights appeared one within the other, the smaller within the larger, the one being the subtle cause and also the support of the other.

One day in meditation I visited a great city. As soon as I saw it, I fell into a deep sleep and so could not see or understand anything about it; I was plunged in its waters of love. I passed through the darkness and reached Tandraloka, where I saw, in the distance, a chariot coming toward me. It was made in a unique way, a way that human ingenuity could not reproduce. It was studded with precious stones, made, not of matter, but of Consciousness. Instead of wheels, it had four small pillars beneath it. It shone all over with rays of divine light, as if illuminated by thousands of suns, and it moved without touching the ground. When I saw it, I was swept away in ecstasy. The chariot approached me and stopped, and a god in human form stepped out. He was dressed in white silk, and wore jeweled sandals on his feet and a girdle around his waist—not like the leather belt that modern men wear, but a belt set with countless jewels. He wore a necklace of pearls, a small jeweled crown on his head, and over his shoulder the sacred thread. His celestial radiance brightened my face and the surrounding mango trees. Luminous rings hung from his ears, and he held a shining weapon in his hand. The god looked at me and smiled, then spoke in Sanskrit, the language of the gods: *rathe upaviśa—* "Sit in the chariot."

I didn't know Sanskrit very well, but somehow I understood him. I immediately got in and sat down. Here another surprise awaited me; from the outside, the chariot looked about ten feet square, but once inside I saw that it was very big and furnished with everything one would need. There was water, a small bathroom, and several bedrooms. The cushions were strangely beautiful. They were set with divine jewels, whose radiance spread light everywhere. There was one seat there which attracted me very much and yet bewildered me.

After he had shown me around, the god took me to an outer room. At that point I felt the chariot setting off at the speed of lightning. I sat down on one seat and looked at the god in human form sitting opposite me on a seat from which two jewels were throwing light on my body. We arrived at a wonderful, extraordinary city, where there were trees bearing blossoms of many colors and divine fragrances, trees laden with many kinds of sweet and juicy fruit, beautiful rippling streams, singing birds, and different kinds of animals. On one side I saw enchanting swans of blue, white, yellow, and black, while on the other, herds of radiant golden deer leaped and bounded fearlessly. Some of them sparkled like diamonds, emeralds, and sapphires. I could also see herds of splendid cows and calves. The winds were laden with divine fragrances. I was in ecstasy at what I saw.

After a time the chariot came to the edge of the city and passed inside it. Everything there was made in a supernatural way, even the bricks, the stones, and the earth. Even the drains were small and beautiful. Truly, this was heaven. The light there was different from that of the sun. The city was illuminated by a silvery light. It was cool; there was no heat. All the leaves of the trees were green, and they did not fade or wither away.

I remind you all that I saw all these scenes in Tandraloka while I was sitting in meditation in my hut in Nagad. Finally we landed near a palace. The paths in front of it were strewn with flowers. Men stood on one side of the path holding garlands, and on the other side stood women holding golden salvers adorned for *arati*. As we both got down from the chariot, they showered me with flowers.

I now understood that the god who was with me was none other than the king of heaven and lord of a hundred sacrifices, Indra himself. He had risen to his present eminence because of the good deeds he had done as a king in a previous life as a human being. Indra is really the king of all worlds. We were both worshiped with *arati*. All the people of the city were young, healthy, and free from sadness. Although their bodies were slim, they were strong, and they all glowed with a remarkable radiance. I had been in Indra's own dwelling place, but now, accompanied by him, I went to see other places and was welcomed in each by *arati*, offered by girls and women, and by flowers strewn on the path. After I had seen everything, we returned to the palace, where a company of classical musicians awaited us. Indraloka is the world of the virtuous, where sensuous desires are fulfilled, and because it grants enjoyment, it may also be called Sakamaloka, the world of the satisfaction of desires. As I looked around, a necklace of pearls and another of flowers were placed over my head. At that moment the flying silver chariot appeared before us. I understood it as a signal for our departure, and Indra and I got in and sat down on our seats. In a short time I was back in Nagad, and my meditation stopped.

I opened my eyes and saw the same scene in front of me. When I shut them I could still see it. I was struck with wonder as I remembered all I had seen. I wandered around a bit outside and my *tandra* trance finally disappeared. I sat down quietly, and thought about everything so that I could remember it all very clearly. In this way the journey of Muktananda's yoga of meditation continued, full of different experiences.

Having seen heaven, hell, and the world of the cobras, I began to have complete faith in the scriptures. Before, I had believed that the only truth was Self-realization and had not believed in heaven, hell, the world of the gods, and other such things. Now I was convinced that what the scriptures said was perfectly true and that it was we who were unable to understand. The ancient sages could see deeply into areas that we cannot see and had composed the scriptures with the omniscience acquired through yoga. This is why their words are true. When we can learn something by doing just a little *sadhana*, how could anything remain hidden from those sages and seers whose *sadhana* was perfect?

Thirteen

Vision of My Own Form

Now I began to have a new experience. As the lights appeared in meditation, I would see myself sitting opposite, even when I opened my eyes. Sometimes, when I had been doing tasks before meditating, I would see myself doing them in meditation. If I had been wandering in the orange orchard, I would see myself strolling here and there. This was another source of wonder for me.

I began to miss Gurudev very much. I wondered when I would go and see him, and when he would call me. As I was feeling this, three dear friends—Nigudkar Guruji, Jivanji Desai, and Babu Shetty—came to see me. They gave me the news from Ganeshpuri, and then I set out to have Gurudev's *darshan*. I stayed in Ganeshpuri for a few days, and then Gurudev told me to go and stay at Gavdevi, in a three-room house that he had had built there. Now that I was living near him, I could go for his *darshan* whenever I felt like it. I went regularly, morning and evening, and sometimes I spent the whole night with him. Sometimes in meditation I would see myself, and at other times, Gurudev. Sometimes, when I sat by the riverside to meditate, I would see myself sitting there. I told Gurudev about this, and he said, "Hmm, good." Later I learned from certain books on yoga that this is called *pratika darsana*, vision of one's own form, and that it is a sign of complete purification of the body. My body was now very thin, but full of energy. I was still meditating. I had completed the meditation on Krishneshwari, the black light, and was now meditating more and more on Neeleshwari, the Blue Pearl. The black light stands for the causal body, which Jnaneshwar Maharaj called *parvardha*—"the tip of a finger." Its seat is in the heart, and in this body deep and dreamless sleep occurs. It is the pure unstained state beyond the senses, and in this state there are no desires, but only the enjoyment of bliss. The individual soul in this body is represented by the "*m*" in *Aum* and is called *prajna.*

Through meditation it is possible to have direct experience of the gross, subtle, causal, and supracausal bodies. The causal body, which I have named Krishneshwari, the black goddess, and which I experienced as the size of a fingertip, is the third petal of the lotus of the four bodies. The first petal is red, the second white, and the third black. Oh Siddha students, you may experience all this for yourselves in meditation. This is something which can be attained only through the regular practice of yoga. The saints have called this *devayana pantha*—"the way of the gods." Kundalini Yoga is the great yoga and the way of God revealed, because in this yoga there is no difference between ordinary life, spiritual life, and God. It is called Siddha Marga, the path of perfection. It is the path to liberation.

The blue *akasha*, an expansion of blue color, began to appear in meditation and with it, the *neela bindu*, the Pearl of infinite power. As I watched it, I felt as if my eyes were going to burst. My eyelids would not move; I could not open or close my eyes. I was completely entranced by the *bindu.* I saw a new light outside also, and as I passed into meditation, Kundalini Mahamaya would appear before me in many different forms. Whatever form She took, I regarded in the same way —as the supreme Shakti, the Goddess Chiti. The Blue Light came and went, came and went. My eyes rolled up so that they were a little above the eyebrows, and apparently lost. Something important was happening in the cranial region. There are some *chakras* there, and this process was happening to purify them.

Now my meditation went beyond the black light to the Blue Pearl. As soon as I sat down to meditate, there would be gentle movement in my body and then a rush of new energy through the *nadis*. The red, white, black, and Blue lights would come. My meditation would stabilize itself, and sometimes I would pass into a deep *tandra* trance and would travel to other worlds. I saw everything while sitting in my hut. Every day I had some new experience. My body was becoming light, slim, agile, healthy, and strong. I could see the central *nadi*, the *sushumna*, which is silver-colored tinged with gold. It stands like a pillar, and all the *nadis* receive vibrations of power from it. When a *sadhaka* is meditating, he sometimes feels a pain in the *muladhara*, at the base of the spine, which is due to the transmission of Shakti from the *sushumna* into the other *nadis*. Sometimes I would have a new movement in the heart, in which an egg-shaped ball of radiance would come into view. This is the vision of the radiant thumb-sized Being, who is described as follows in the *Shvetashvatara Upanishad: aṅguṣṭhamātraḥ puruṣo'ntarātmā sadā janānāṁ hridaye sanniviṣṭaḥ*—"The inner soul always dwells in the heart of all men as a thumb-sized being."

Fifteen

The World of Omniscience

Next, I saw a light that was different from the red, white, black and Blue lights, and as it came into view, I saw many, many worlds within it. It was a soft saffron color, and in the middle of it were thousands of soft blue sparks and a soft golden radiance. It was very sweet and lovely. It arose within the series of four lights that I had already experienced. I saw many clairvoyant visions in this new light, so I watched it with great attention. Just as I had habitually passed into Tandraloka in meditation, so I now entered the place within the radiant light. I shall call it Sarvajnaloka, the world of omniscience. The great Indian seers and sages who attained this place through the yoga of meditation became omniscient, and if they wanted to, they could go there even in the waking state. Through the grace of Parashakti, a *sadhaka* will occasionally reach this state in meditation. When my mind became stabilized in Sarvajnaloka, I could see far away into many different worlds. Everything I saw there was perfectly genuine. Sometimes I would see some accident in the outside world—a factory catching fire or a river in flood—and these things always actually happened. However, it was only through the grace of the Goddess Chiti that I could visit Sarvajnaloka in meditation and see all these things. I could not see them whenever I wanted. I saw many marvelous scenes in meditation.

Some yogis acquire *siddhis*, or supernatural powers, from Sarvajnaloka. Through meditation one can very soon get ordinary *siddhis*, but the highest aspirant, being a true child of his Guru, longs only for perfection. He doesn't care at all for these powers, and he doesn't tell other people about any powers he may acquire. Students of meditation! Your duty is to honor and respect the Shakti of the Guru's grace, which you can feel active within you, by loving the Guru. Always be aware of your own importance, your own depth, your own faith, and your own holy bodies.

Every day I meditated on the Blue Pearl and had many visions. While I was having this joyful meditation on Neeleshwari, I started to hear music in my inner ear. I heard it first in my left ear. In some book or other it says that, if the *nada*, the divine music, is heard first in the left ear, then one is about to die. Several friends warned me solemnly about this, but I replied that death comes at its own particular time, appointed by destiny, and I kept on with my meditation. I meditated on the Blue Pearl with great love. Besides this music, I began to hear a very fine and subtle sound, still in my left ear. Now I was watching the lights and listening to the sounds, and my meditation became even more intense. I heard the fine, mellow sound of the strings of the *veena*.

One day I wanted to ask Gurudev about the *nada*. I always went at the same time every day for his *darshan*, but that day I went at a different time. I stood in front of him, knowing that that great omniscient sage would shake his head and ask, "What?"—which is what happened. His head was swaying, and he was making his little humming sounds. I said, "Baba, people say that when you hear the *nada* in your left ear you will die." Babaji said, "What's left? What's right? They're both God's. Yes. Both ears belong to God. You don't hear the *nada* in the ear, but in the inner ear, in the inner space." It is quite true that that *nada* does not come from the right or left ear, nor from in front or behind. It is the sweet, divine music of the gods reverberating in the inner space; it is the sound of the *chidakasha*, the space of Consciousness. It is not an ominous foreboding of death but the mantra of the original vibrations of Chiti, the most subtle vibratory level of speech, which leads one to Godhood. Yogis and *jnanis* can discover the source of their being through this sound. Jnaneshwar Maharaj said: *nādāchīye pailatīrīṁ turīyāchiye mājhe ghar*—"On the yonder shore, across the *nada*, is my abode of *turiya.*" Such a sublime and auspicious *nada* cannot be an omen of death; it is the herald of immortal life.

I was now seeing the miracles of Chiti within the Blue Pearl as well as listening to the *nada*. I meditated every day; indeed, I could not find enjoyment in anything other than meditation. Once in meditation my eyes rolled upward, became inverted, and stayed in that position. I saw a firmament filled with white lights and heard divine sounds all around. My mind became concentrated on this, and I saw an extremely beautiful, shining blue star. It was not the Blue Pearl, but it was marvelously brilliant. It looked just like the familiar planet Venus, which we can see shining in the west in the evening, and in the east at daybreak. This beautiful star is located in the center of the upper space of the *sahasrara*, and it never moves. I watched it for the whole of my meditation. When I came out of *tandra,* I got up and began to walk about outside. I went up onto the hill behind the Gavdevi temple, wondering what the star could have been. I was sitting on the part of the hill where there now stands the Turiya Mandir of Shree Gurudev Ashram. It was all forest then, and I sometimes used to sit alone up there till 8:00 or 9:00 at night. That night, as I was sitting there, a star descended from the sky and disappeared. It was just like the star I had seen in meditation. I was puzzled by this and did not understand it at all. I started to meditate again, and felt waves of rapture and delight and love flow within me. I went on meditating, and the firmament appeared again with the star shining steadily.

My meditation became more and more subtle. At this stage, meditating yogis have to be extremely careful. Through the vision of the Blue Pearl they will certainly achieve liberation, but they will not be able to attain complete realization of Godhead; their experience will only be partial. For full realization one has to enter within the Blue Pearl to the inner Self. It is, of course, true that the dawning of the Blue Pearl brings great peace. If a seeker does not get to see the Blue Pearl, his condition will be like that of an ignorant man who does not see the soul, but only the body.

A traveler on the path of realization experiences the Self as a living reality. Sri Tukaram, that blessed jewel among saints who attained full realization of God, says in one of his immortal verses:

> *tira evaḍheṁ bāndhūni ghara*
> *āṁta rāhe viśvaṁbhara*

tiṛā ituke biṅdule
teṇeṁ tribhuvana koṅdātale
harïharāchyā mūrti
biṅdulyāṁta yetï jātï
tukā mhaṇe he biṅdule
teṇeṁ tribhuvana koṅdātale

Tukaram Maharaj says in this verse that God, the Nourisher of the universe, lives in a house as tiny as a sesame seed. He is called the Nourisher because He sustains the whole universe. The Lord of the universe, the supreme Self of all living beings, the power of *prana*, who is known inwardly through the higher intuition by yogis, devotees, and *jnanis*, who is the treasure-house of omniscience, has made His dwelling place a house as small as a sesame seed. Just as a huge spreading tree grows from a tiny seed, the Nourisher of all, who manifests Himself in an infinity of forms, shapes, and sizes, has a tiny seed for a house. The tiny seed is the source of the huge tree, the tree is contained in the seed, but the seed has a separate existence as a seed. One seed can grow into a tree, and the tree gives birth to countless seeds that are essentially the same as the first; in the same way, the *bindu*, the divine seed, can manifest in endless ways and forms and yet preserve its original identity. The Lord who lives in the *bindu* never loses His integrity nor His original power. His greatness and glory remain complete and unchanging.

This can be made clearer by another analogy. We know that man is born of a man and that he has all the characteristics of his progenitor. A son is born from one drop of his father's semen, but the father does not lose anything of himself when the son is born; he stays the same as before in all respects, and the son born from his father's semen is as complete as his father. His physical characteristics are like his father's, and so also is his way of behaving. We can say that the father is reborn as his son and that the son is therefore not a son, but the father. In the same manner, God, the source of the universe, creates the infinite universe within His own being by activating the Chitshakti in His own Self. He pervades it and yet transcends it. In other words, He builds His house within His own being and lives in it. Tukaram Maharaj's lines: *tilā evaḍhe bandhūni ghara ānta rāhe viśvambhara*—"The

Nourisher of the universe lives in a house as tiny as a sesame seed," are perfectly true, and there can be no doubt or argument about them.

The *bindu*, which is as small as a sesame seed, is the house of the Self. God is inside it—God who is the perfect form of the Self. If you have a vision of the *bindu*, then you should understand that within it lies your Self. It is this *bindu* I have called Neeleshwari, the Blue Goddess, the Blue Pearl. This Pearl is as big as a sesame seed and like a house, and the supreme Self, God, lives in that house. Tukaram says that this *bindu* in fact contains the three worlds within it. Just think—heaven, the human world, and hell are all inside it.

The individual soul is enclosed within four bodies, one within the other, which I have called the red, the white, the black, and the blue. The red corresponds to the gross body, the white to the subtle body, the black to the causal body, and the blue to the supracausal body. The supracausal body is within the Blue Pearl. Through meditation you can fully realize how the three worlds can be contained within a *bindu* as small as a sesame seed. Furthermore, Tukaram says, "The trinity of Brahma, Vishnu, and Shiva come and go within the *bindu*." This *bindu* is the dwelling place of these three gods. Siddha students, now you can understand for yourselves how great, how significant, how sublime is the tiny *bindu* that you see in meditation. God, the supporter of the three worlds, lives within you in the tiny Blue Pearl. Therefore, O man, seek Him within you in reverence for God and in the company of great beings. Until you have searched within, what can you possibly see? You may have seen Paris, London, and New York, but you have only seen a fraction of just this one world. Yet the Lord dwells within you with His three worlds. These things are not meant just to be talked about or heard, they are meant to be attained, and through steadfast practice they will be attained.

The Blue Pearl is a great and holy pilgrimage center. Jnaneshwar Maharaj says:

> *doṛāṅchī pāhā doṛāṁ śūnyāchā śevaṭa*
> *nīṛa biṅdū nīṭa lakhalakhīta*

The eye of the eye, the *neelabindu*, even beyond the void, is brilliant and sparkling.

This radiant and scintillating and sublime Blue Pearl can be seen directly in meditation. O Siddha students, you can have *darshan* of it! But you have to remember that, if you want to see such a great and wonderful thing, your way of life and your habits must be the purest and the most holy. You have to become worthy of it. Your associations, your words, and your thoughts should be full of God. He who has seen the Blue Pearl is the most blessed of all human beings. It is written in the *Skanda Purana*:

> *kulaṁ pavitraṁ jananī kṛutārthā vasundharā puṇyavatī cha tena*
> *apārasaṁvitsukhasāgare'smīnllīnaṁ pare brahmaṇi yasya chetaḥ*

> The whole family of a *sadhaka* in whom Chiti is flourishing becomes holy, because the Shakti makes everything holy. The mother of such a boy or girl herself becomes fulfilled. The earth upon which he walks becomes holy.

Only the family in which such pure souls are born is truly noble. The houses of the men and women or boys and girls in whom the Shakti is awake and blossoming are equal to all holy places of pilgrimage; let there be no doubt about this. The minds of these souls whose inner Shakti is continually expanding become absorbed in the limitless universal Consciousness, the Absolute, the ocean of bliss. All holy rivers merge at the place where the students of the yoga of meditation live. They themselves are sacred, and to have their *darshan* is itself a good and beneficial thing.

> In the *Srimad Bhagavatam* (11:14:24), the Lord says:

> *vāggadgadā dravate yasya chittaṁ rudatyabhīkshaṇaṁ hasati*
> *   kvachichcha*
> *vilajja udgāyati ṇrutyate cha madbhaktiyukto bhuvanaṁ punāti*

> His mind melts with choking words. He weeps at every moment; sometimes he laughs. He sings loudly and dances without shame. One devoted to Me sanctifies the world.

Divine love is revealed in the man whose inner Shakti has been awakened by the power of the Guru's grace. His voice becomes so filled with joy that when he speaks he scatters love. His mind is always melting with love; he weeps again and again in a frenzy of love; sometimes he abandons all shame and starts to dance and sing loudly. When a *sadhaka* of Siddha Yoga becomes such a great lover of God, he can sanctify the three worlds. When the supremely ecstatic Chiti begins Her work and when one has the vision of the Blue Pearl, this love arises from within. It is this love that overwhelms the tongue and melts the mind. A student can then purify all his four bodies through meditation. He makes every place where he meditates a holy place. By his presence, such a devotee sanctifies even the holy centers of pilgrimage. Because the vibrations of Chiti in his heart appear in his words, his words are scripture and prove the truth of the scriptures. He makes all actions—his own and other peoples'—beneficial, for since all his actions are inspired by Chiti, whatever he does brings good. Everything turned out well for anyone who was blessed by my Gurudev; even those whom he abused became famous. This is how it is when Chiti inspires everything men do. Chiti flows from their left over food. Even in their bathrooms there are thick concentrations of the Chiti of all blessings.

Once while I was writing this book, a strong wave of Shakti seized my body. I asked a young college student, who had recently come and was standing nearby, to massage my head a little, as it was feeling rather heavy. He did this, and even while he was standing there, the Chiti Shakti entered his body and he received divine Shaktipat. He started to assume the *maha mudra* and other *mudras*, and he reached a high state of yoga. Such is the unbounded glory of Chiti. Only he who has experienced it for himself can believe or understand it. If a man's heart has been destroyed and his mind has been warped and corrupted, what can this ignorant person know of the power and mysteries of Chiti? The Mother has created this peerless and beautiful universe out of nothing and with the help of no one, so what can She not achieve through the Guru?

I am going to tell you something rather interesting. I have a very beautiful and well-kept bathroom. Not only do I not let anyone else bathe there, but I do not even let anyone else clean it, except for my dear disciple Venkappa, who was initiated many years ago. Yogis who give Shaktipat must have pure and beautiful bathrooms. We used to drink my Gurudev's bathwater as holy water because it was saturated with rays of Chiti. No one is ever allowed into my bathroom. One day a dear student of Siddha Yoga, an officer with an airline company, begged for permission to clean it, so I said, "Go ahead." While he was cleaning it he sat down and stayed there for four hours. The rays of Chiti permeating the bathroom had fallen on him; they had entered him, and he had received Shaktipat. He sat in *samadhi* for four hours. I thought to myself, "He hasn't come out yet," and went in to find him in the lotus posture, lost in ecstasy. I interrupted his *samadhi*, made him get up, and brought him outside. Now people fall into meditation in his meditation room.

The reason I write this is to show that Chiti Shakti is always flowing from the bodies of Siddha students. Rays of Chiti were constantly flowing from my Guru, whatever he was doing. When a ray struck another person, that person would begin to have divine experiences. Everything that a Siddha does is motivated by Chiti Shakti. If he merely touches someone with his finger, Shakti will enter him. Anybody who is touched by a Siddha's body receives Shakti, and anybody who wears a Siddha's old clothes will be entered by Shakti. Siddha students, whatever place you meditate in, you make a house of God. The place where you live becomes a great holy place. Holy places take their holiness from you. The mantra becomes enlivened from you. The various aspects of yoga—*asanas, mudras, pranayama*, and so on—practiced by followers of external yoga take place automatically in people by your touch. Your very breathing is priceless. Remember always that rays of Chiti stream from the hairs of your body. You must realize that you yourselves are fields of Chiti where the greatest goddess of all, the deity most worthy of adoration, Mother Chiti Shakti, has become incarnated in Her dynamic form. The Guru himself sits within you all as the power of divine grace. Don't think you are small, don't think you are stupid, don't think you are too young or too dependent on others. The One from whom this world takes its being, the One who is Herself the very form of the world, the same Goddess Chiti in whom the world is fulfilled, can be directly experienced within your own Self. This is why you are the holiest of holy places, the mantra of mantras, the god of gods, and the holy essence of worship. You should understand how worthy you really are, keep silent as much as possible, be pure in mind, and lead a life of good conduct and devotion. Don't let yourself get involved in artificial and impure ways.

One more thing I want to remind you about: expulsion of faeces is far better than discharge of seminal fluid. This is not just for *sadhus*, renunciants, and celibates, because they have no relationship with the world anyway. It is for worldly people. You should live in the world and be happy. Husband and wife should look upon each other as gods and love each other very much. You should preserve your seminal fluid, which is your radiance, as you save money, watching every penny. Never forget that a radiant human being can be formed from one drop of semen. Remember the value of the radiance of that one drop. If you lose it, all the best powders and creams and rouges and lipsticks will not brighten your skin. The radiance of the sexual fluid is the vehicle of Chiti Shakti. Chiti is, as it were, bought with it. It is the means for activating the Kundalini and the highest means of making *samadhi* stable. Look carefully and see the condition of the man who has wasted his sexual fluid.

My dear Siddha students, listen to what I say. You are the very incarnation of Chiti. You should realize that it is your true reality, and so keep yourselves pure. One drop of the same light that lives within you can make the sun, the moon, and the stars. With just a little *sadhana* you can reach the stage where Chiti Shakti flows into others just through your touch or even your company. Even this is a lot. When you become worthy of the Guru's grace and can activate the vibrations of Shakti in other people through the radiance attained in only a short period of *sadhana*, think how much worth you will have after you have practiced *sadhana* properly and truly for a long time. You can become so great! Why should the world not worship you as an ideal father or mother?

Here is a warning for Siddha students. It is very good that you have accumulated so much Shakti through meditation in a very short period of purity, but you can lose this Shakti before you have stored up the maximum amount. You have to look after it. You must be vigilant while standing, sitting, coming, going, giving, taking, and in anything you do. Increase your store of Chiti rather than decreasing it. You should not undermine your *sadhana* by listening to the opinions of evil, leering types of people whose minds are perverted and whose habits are bad. If you do find yourself in the company of some hypocrite who distorts everything, then spit in his face, close your eyes and pray, "O Sadguru, you are the father of all. You are my mother. Save me." If you remain vigilant, your *sadhana* will progress quickly. I am describing the greatness of the Siddha student because his worth increases after he begins to see the Blue Pearl in meditation. In this connection let me give the meaning of one of Jnaneshwar's verses. Remember it. Jnaneshwar says, "I shall dwell at the feet of him who sees the Being who lives between the eyebrows. I shall always meditate on the nature of him who secretly sees the divine Blue Light, which lives between the eyebrows. O people! He who sees the Blue in the space between the eyebrows, he alone is blessed, he alone is fortunate."

There is another verse by Jnaneshwar that I very much like to give—it is like a deity which I worship. It is a great mantra not only for me, but for all those on the path to liberation. Furthermore, what I am going to quote is a testimony of my own inner experience, it is the criterion of realization and the key to the mystery of the Guru. This is why I regard this verse as a mantra. O my dear Siddha students, listen! Read it carefully, as it contains the mystery of mysteries:

> *dorāṅchi pāhā dorāṁ śūnyāchā śevaṭa*
> *nīra bindū nīṭa lakhalakhīta*
> *visāvoṁ āleṁ pātaleṁ chaitanya tetheṁ*
> *pāhe pā nirūteṁ anubhaveṁ*
> *pārvatīlāgiṁ ādīnātheṁ dāvileṁ*
> *jñānadevā phāvaleṁ nivrittikripā*

> O seekers after the knowledge of perfection, the very eye of your eye, where the void comes to an end, the Blue Pearl, pure, sparkling, radiant, that which opens the center of repose when it arises, is the great place of the conscious Self. Look, my brother, this is the hidden secret of this experience. This is what Parashiva, the primal Lord, told Parvati. Jnanadeva says, 'I saw this through the grace of my Sadguru Nivrittinath.'

Such is the significance of the *neela bindu*, which I have called Neeleshwari, the Blue Goddess. Just from seeing this Blue Pearl you can attain *jivanmukti*, the state of liberation. But this is not full realization, nor the state of perfection, nor the final goal of the Siddha Path. When you see the Blue Pearl all the time, this means that you are in the *turiya* state, the state of complete transcendence. If a seeker dies after having this vision, he will go to Brahmaloka, the world of Brahman, and attain complete fulfillment by finishing his *sadhana* there.

Now I often saw a wonderfully luminous ball of light. It was much brighter than the other lights, and as I gazed at it, my meditation became better and better. As before, the four lights would appear first of all, and when the Blue Pearl appeared, my mind would converge on it for long periods of time, experiencing extremely joyful repose. My breathing became steady and shallow. When I breathed out, the breath would go only the distance of about two fingers from my nostrils, and when I breathed in, it would go down only as far as my throat, never to my heart. However, I did not pay much attention to this for fear that my meditation would be disturbed; I always took great care that my meditation should remain firm. During this stage, many divine fragrances came to me. They were so fine that compared with them even the finest scents brought to me by my dear devotees were dull and flat. There is no fragrance in the world to equal these divine fragrances, and they made me quite drunk. I floated in ecstasy—they were so divine. The experience stayed with me for a long time. With the coming of these fragrances, my breathing became very short and slow, and a special kind of *pranayama* took place spontaneously. When my breathing was like this, there arose in me the most sweet and beautiful love. It felt like a direct, true revelation of God. Love is God. That is why Narada says in the *Bhakti Sutras* (51): *anirvachaniyam premasvarūpam*—"Love is indescribable in its very nature."

With these experiences of the subtle levels, my enjoyment of meditation increased and increased. My mind was in such an extraordinary state that in every meditation I felt great joy and rapture, and every day this rapture increased so that the bliss of the day before seemed as nothing. I discovered that there is no limit to this kind of joy. Love grows steadily deeper, and there is no final point to love.

With this experience I came to understand that there was still something ahead. Sometimes in meditation everything would abruptly change. My eyes would slowly roll up and become centered on the upper space of the *sahasrara*. Instead of seeing two images separately, my eyes saw one. This is what is called *bindu bheda*. Ah! What a great gift of Siddha Yoga! How mighty the power of Kundalini! What is understood intellectually through books and study can be experienced directly through Siddha Yoga.

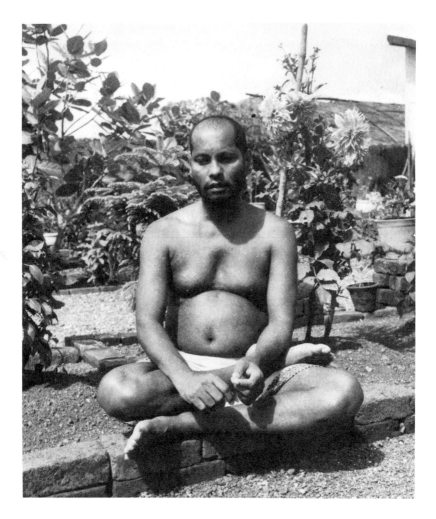

Swami Muktananda in his garden at Ganeshpuri, 1959

Sixteen

Visit to the World
of the Siddhas

Again the blue star shone steadily before me, not moving at all. While I gazed within at the upper regions of the *sahasrara*, I traveled to many worlds with the blue star as my vehicle. It was not the Blue Light or the Blue Pearl, but a blue star. Though it looked small, it was large enough to contain me. One day it took me far away, and set me down in the most beautiful world, the most entrancing of all those I had seen. I cannot describe its beauty, for words would be an insult to it. In this world I came upon a fascinating path, and, following it, I saw many woods, caves both large and small, flowing streams of pure water, white, blue, and green deer, and also some white peacocks. The atmosphere was very calm and peaceful, and there was a beautiful blue light everywhere, such as you would see if you looked at the early morning sun through a piece of blue glass. There was no sun or moon, only light spreading everywhere. When I arrived I felt such strong waves and impulses of Shakti that I knew intuitively that I was going to have the *darshan* of the ancient seers. I started to move around with the speed of thought. And then what? This was Siddhaloka, the world of the Siddhas! I saw many Siddhas, all of them deeply absorbed in meditation. Each one was in a different *mudra*. None of them looked at me. Some had long, matted hair, some were clean-shaven, and some had pierced ears. Some were sitting under trees, some were sitting on stones, and some were inside caves. I also saw the great seers I had read about in the *Puranas*. I saw Sai Baba of Shirdi. Though Nityananda

Baba was in Ganeshpuri, he was here, too. Each Siddha had his own hut or cave or house made in styles I had never seen. Some of the Siddhas were just sitting quietly.

The climate was very good and the light very pleasing. I found that I now knew everything. I recognized the seers and sages of ancient times and, moving on a little, saw many yoginis, all sitting steadily in their various divine *mudras*. I spent a long time wandering around Siddhaloka looking at the yoginis and Siddha saints. I was very fascinated by Siddhaloka. No other world had seemed so good to me. I did not feel like leaving and thought it would be very nice if I could stay. Then I saw a huge lotus pond with golden lotuses growing in it. Turning away from this pond, I saw the Seven Sages in a group, a sight which brought me peace, happiness, and love. I went on roaming in this state of peace and love; it seemed that someone unknown was guiding me. I entered another forest—very beautiful. I did not recognize the species of any trees in it. I saw more Siddhas there and felt the desire, as I had earlier, to sit down in the lotus posture and meditate. As soon as I sat, the blue star appeared, and for some reason I felt compelled to go and sit in it. I don't know how I did this or who was controlling me. Anyway, the star at once took me back at immense speed to the place where I was meditating.

When I arrived, the blue star passed within me into my *sahasrara* and exploded. Its fragments spread throughout the vast spaces of the *sahasrara*. There was no star in front of me now, but just an ambrosial white light. Then I passed into Tandraloka, which was quite near to me. At that moment a Siddha, whom I did not know, appeared to me from Siddhaloka and said, "You have just seen Siddhaloka, the world of the Siddhas. Here live the great saints who have achieved *jivanmukti*, liberation. There is no hunger, no sleep, and no awakening. One eats joy, drinks joy, lives in joy, and continually experiences joy. Everything there is joy. Just as a fish sleeps in water, lives in water, eats in water, and plays in water, so the inhabitants of Siddhaloka abide in joy. Without the grace of a Siddha, no one can go there. Those who are doing the *sadhana* of the Siddha Path, who belong to the Siddha tradition, and who will attain full Siddhahood will go to Siddhaloka. The blue star, which became your vehicle and took you there, is the only way of traveling to it. It can also take you to other worlds. But until the star explodes, the cycle of birth and rebirth is not broken, the bondage to *karma* is not cut, the veil of sins and good deeds is not torn away. Only when that is torn is the eye of differentiation removed." After he said this and blessed me, the saint disappeared.

Seventeen

A Golden Lotus
Falls on My Head

I was in Tandraloka, in great exultation and excitement, and a shower of flowers was falling on my head. As the flowers fell, my attention was drawn upward. I saw the same Siddha. From the lake in Siddhaloka he was hurling a golden lotus about two feet across. I watched it coming down, and as it fell, there was a soft humming sound of the chanting of *Om*. It hit my head with tremendous force and made an audible thud. When I heard this sound my eyes opened, but I was still in Tandraloka. It was as if someone had given me a hard slap on the head. I could see the golden lotus lying on the ground where it had fallen after it had hit my head. How beautiful it was, how amazingly well-formed, and what a fine scent was coming from it! I went on looking at it with surprise and curiosity. I was watching it, congratulating myself on my good fortune, and marveling at the magnificence of the lotus, when I suddenly remembered my Gurudev's grace. I quickly closed my eyes and inwardly bowed to him. When I opened my eyes again, the lotus was no longer there. How strange it was. What had happened? What an amazing experience. My mind was filled with these questions. I can still feel the impact of the lotus as it struck my head. I undid my legs from the meditation posture. The meditation period was now over, and I went outside and wandered around for a bit. I looked at the sky for a moment. I bowed in the direction of my Gurudev, in Ganeshpuri. I sat peacefully in the orchard. I closed my eyes again and thought of what I had seen and experienced in meditation and visualized those scenes again.

Later when I sat to meditate, there were first some physical *kriyas* and then the red aura. If I do not always mention this red light, the reader should nevertheless not forget it, for just as day begins with sunrise, so meditation begins with the dawning of the red aura. Its brilliance increased all the time so that it was no longer the same as when it had first appeared; now it shone with a truly divine radiance. I supposed this was due to the mingling of its light with that of the blue star, which had burst and spread throughout the *sahasrara*. Or perhaps it was because of my vision of Siddhaloka. Why not? It was quite likely. If I went to Benares, I would earn some merit; if I went to Dwarka or Rameshwaram, I would bring back some reward; if I went to Ganeshpuri, I would experience some joy—so why should I not get something from my journey to Siddhaloka? Then I thought about the golden lotus that had fallen on my head, and thought, "I have just returned from Siddhaloka and after that the golden lotus struck my head. Maybe everything has happened because of its touch."

Inside the red aura thousands of sparks from the exploded star twinkled. By their light I could see within me all my nerves, my excretory system, my gall bladder, and my internal organs. Inside the red aura I then saw a beautiful light moving with great speed. It was the light of my Sadguru's power of grace. As I watched, the red aura disappeared and was followed by the thumb-sized white flame. It too shone with a new and ever-increasing luster. Then the black light appeared inside the white light, also shining more brightly, and finally there came the Blue Pearl, streaming with the rays of a new radiance. The Pearl was still blue, but was much brighter than before; its brilliance was increasing every day. My mind became absorbed in this tremendous radiance, and with this absorption a very high state of love began to flow in my heart. This love was as all-pervasive as the rays of blue light spreading through all my *nadis*, and like the light, its waves and eddies jumped and played in the *nadis*. I also felt its vibrations in my sense organs. Waves of Chiti and waves of ecstasy spread all through me. As I meditated in these raptures of love, I would pass into Tandraloka.

Once while I was in Tandraloka, the secret of my vision of Siddhaloka was revealed to me. Siddhaloka is perfectly real and exists for anyone who attains perfection, whatever his religion. The golden lotus that fell on my head was a gift, a blessing full of divine grace, from Siddhaloka. The blue star in which I had traveled is found in the *sahasrara* of every creature. Its brilliance can vary, but its size is the same. And it is also by means of this star that the individual soul passes from one body to another in the cycle of birth and rebirth. However many times a man is burned or buried, the blue star will always stay the same. It leaves the body at death, but stays at the place of death for eleven days. Afterward, according to destiny, it carries the soul with its sins and virtues to different worlds. The blue star is the self-propelled vehicle of the individual soul. When the individual is born again, the blue star is born with it. When the star exploded, my cycle of coming and going was ended. The vehicle had broken down, so how could I come and go any more? This breaking may also be called the piercing of the knot of the heart. In Tandraloka I learned that all the *karma* of my previous births had been cancelled out, and as I learned this, the whole world immediately changed for me. All these experiences were not under my control but under the control of the inner Shakti, because the Shakti is completely independent.

Eighteen

The World of Ancestors

While describing my experiences, I have left out one that is very important and should be told, namely, my visit to the world of ancestors. This world is situated between heaven and Siddhaloka, and many categories of ancestors are to be found there. I have actually seen them. In heaven, in the world of cobras, and in the world of the moon, everyone has the same enjoyments and pleasures, but here they do not. There are the rich, the virtuous, the moderately rich, the less virtuous, and the poor—the same kinds of inequalities that we find on earth. Nonetheless, people are happier there than they are here. In Pitruloka I saw some old people I had known in childhood. It is a unique world. There can be no doubt that the various ritual offerings of water and foodstuffs that we make to our ancestors do actually reach them in a subtle form. It is true that they eat what we give them, that they accept our offerings and give their blessings to their descendants, so we should please them by giving them offerings. O Siddha students, you should not have the slightest doubt about this. The subtle form of the offering reaches the world of the ancestors through the mantras we repeat. The same Chiti Shakti carries it from here to there by means of the mantras. Let me give an example from life today. Suppose you have a friend in America. America is very far from here, but he can tell you on the telephone that he has sent you many dollars through his bank and that you can get them here. You will certainly get the money. This is only a material transaction carried out through physical sound over a telephone—this is something you all know. So why should you doubt that the subtle forms of the offerings are carried to the world of ancestors through mantras?

In Pitruloka I saw many people. I had traveled there in the same blue star in which I had visited Siddhaloka. I remind you again that it was not the Blue Pearl or the Blue Light, but the blue star. O Siddha students, the world you and I live in is Mrityuloka, the world of mortals. The world of the ancestors is as real as the mortal world; I have seen it with my own eyes. This reminds me of a story about Eknath Maharaj. I used to doubt the truth of this story, though actually it is not a good thing to question the character of great saints nor their high qualities and deeds. I had picked up my doubts from the wrong sort of company, but as I have already said, one should not have any doubts about the ways and habits of Siddhas or try to judge the rightness or wrongness of their actions. Everything they do is a holy ritual because everything they do is divinely inspired. Sri Eknath Maharaj could see everything. He had attained complete realization of God and saw the one supreme divine Self in forests and towns, in high and low, in what was acceptable and what was rejectable, in sinners and the virtuous, for the eye of a Siddha does not see name, form, and shape, but only the true reality. I shall first illustrate this by another story.

There was once a shepherd called Ramja, who was very rich. He had a golden statue of his deity, Khandoba, and his mount for worship. The mount was a horse, and this image was bigger than that of the god. What the great saints say is quite true: Lakshmi, the goddess of fortune, is fickle, and there is nothing that lasts. Times are always changing, and Ramja's condition also changed. He was rich, but he became poor. You may understand it like this: a mother has two children—one called wealth, the other called poverty—and they are true brothers. In the same way, pleasure and pain, fame and disgrace, live together like brothers. They love each other very much, and so they never live far from each other and never forget each other. Sometimes the elder brother welcomes us, and sometimes the younger. When the elder brother welcomes us we get wealth, power, prosperity, and a kingdom. When the younger says to the elder, "Brother, rest for a while; I'll serve now," then we get want, beggary, misfortune, and misery.

This is exactly what happened to Ramja. The elder brother went away for a rest and the younger came to greet him. He lost everything and could hardly find the money to eat and drink. People said to him, "O Ramja, why do you let yourself suffer so much? Why don't you take the gold statues in your shrine, ask the Lord's forgiveness, and sell them? Then you can get more sheep and start up your work again. You will be able to save money, and then you can get new images, have them installed, worship them, and hold a feast for *brahmins, sadhus,* and the poor, the blind and the lame. When your work goes well, you will be able to perform good deeds."

When man becomes poor, even his thoughts become poor like the younger brother; poverty is not only of riches, but also of thoughts. Ramja agreed to what the people were saying, and he wrapped his Khandoba and the horse in a cloth and went to the goldsmith's market. He sat down in a goldsmith's shop. The goldsmith said, "Hello, Ramja, what's the matter?"

Ramja unwrapped the images of Lord Khandoba and his horse from the cloth and said, "I want to sell these. I need money to live, so I have to sell them. Tell me what they're worth." The goldsmith weighed them. The image of Lord Khandoba weighed one kilo, and that of the horse three kilos. In those days one used to get a kilo of gold for only a thousand *rupees.* The goldsmith said, "Ramja, I'll give you a thousand *rupees* for the god, and three thousand for the horse."

At this, Ramja lost his temper. "Listen, don't you have any brains?" he cried. "A thousand for my Lord and three thousand for His horse! Don't you understand anything?" Ramja got red with anger.

The goldsmith said, "Listen Ramja, you're the one with no brains. You see them as the Lord and His horse, but to me they are just gold, and they are worth what they weigh. Your god is a kilo of gold; so it's worth a thousand *rupees.* Your horse is three kilos of gold; so it's worth three thousand. If you want to sell them, sell them; otherwise be on your way."

The great Siddha Eknath Maharaj had equality of vision like this. He would see only the gold; for him there was only God everywhere in the world. He had no awareness of higher and lower, of differences between castes, between individuals, between great and small. *Harireva jagat*—"The Lord Himself is the universe" was the way he saw it, and he lived in a spirit of complete equality. One day, a girl from the *mahar* caste, who are untouchables, came to see him, and spoke to him with great love and affection, "O Baba, God draws water for you at your house. I can't see that God, nor can I call Him. O Eknath Baba, you are my God. Please come to my hut and eat my plain dry bread and chutney. I have heard your stories. You say that a great saint is just like God. So, Baba, please come and eat at my house. I have come to invite you." In this way she very humbly invited him, and Eknath Maharaj accepted. He went to her house and ate the simple food she prepared for him. All the people saw him. And then what happened? They all started talking about it.

People said, "Look at that Eknath; he's a *brahmin* and a devout worshiper of Vishnu, and he had a meal at an untouchable's house. Shame on him. He has become defiled. No *brahmin* will go to the house of this man who has broken the *dharma* of his caste." So all the *brahmins* of the town excommunicated him.

This made no difference to Eknath Maharaj. He was as happy and joyful as ever. It was his way to welcome good and bad fortune as the same, so he was quite unperturbed. The whole village turned against him, saying things about him, insulting him, and condemning what he had done. But Eknath Maharaj did not suffer at all. Though he was a householder, this great saint had an outlook of complete equality:

mamatā nahīṁ sutadāra meṁ nahīṁ deha meṁ abhimāna hai
nindā praśansā eka sī sama māna arū apamāna hai
jo bhoga āte bhogatā hotā na viṣayāsakta hai
nirvāsanā nirdvandva so ichchhā vinā hī muktā hai
saba viśva apanā jānatā yā kuchha na apanā mānatā
kyā mitra ho kyā śatru saba ko eka sama sanmānatā
sab viśva kā hai bhakta jo sab viśva jiskā bhakta hai
nirhetu sabkā suhrid so ichchhā binā hī mukta hai
māyā nahīṁ kāyā nahīṁ bandhyā rachā yaha viśva hai
nahīṁ nāma hī nahīṁ rūpa hī kevala ika īśa hī paripūrṇa hai
jo īśvara hai vahī jīva hai vahī saba jaga kā paramātma tattva hai
aisā jise nishchaya huā vaha ichchhā binā hī mukta hai

Unattached to his wife and children, not having pride in
    the body,
Accepting praise or blame, honor or insult equally,
Enjoying pleasures as they come, but not indulging in them,
Without longing or conflict, without desire, he is liberated.
Either accepting the entire universe or nothing as his own,
Honoring everyone, friend or foe alike;
Worshiping the whole universe, worshiped by the whole
    universe,
Wishing everyone well without selfish motive, without desire,
    he is liberated.
Neither *maya* nor the body exists. The universe is unreal,
    like a barren woman's child.
Names and forms do not exist. God alone is complete in
    His fullness.
The individual Self is the same as the universal Self. God is
    the divine essence of the world.
Holding this conviction, without desire, he is liberated.

In this way Eknath Maharaj was always free and joyful. Every day there were religious discussions, devotional singing, and meditation on God at his house. He sat in bliss, rose in bliss, and slept in bliss. God is bliss. The world He made is full of joy, as He is. To be able to see the blissful nature of the world is a gift of the Guru's grace. Eknath Maharaj used to live like this, in bliss and freedom of spirit.

A few days after this had happened to Eknath Maharaj, the yearly fortnight sacred to the ancestors came. As I have already said, our offerings really reach our ancestors in Pitruloka, and so it is necessary to make offerings to them. We, their children, are greatly indebted to them. We should never forget that our parents gave us their vital fluids, their blood, and even their food. They do not think of eating, but of giving food to their children; they do not think of sleeping, but of letting their children sleep. Anything special that comes their way, they give to their children to eat, and then they eat what's left. What don't parents do for their children? This is why we are always indebted to our ancestors. It is essential for a virtuous son to make offerings to his ancestors at this time. According to the religious tradition, *brahmins, sannyasis*, and other guests are invited and feasted courteously during this special fortnight, and offerings are made to the ancestors. At this time Eknath Maharaj also invited all the *brahmins* to eat. But because Eknath had eaten at the untouchable girl's house, no *brahmin* came. So Eknath Maharaj invoked the ancestors, and the dead fathers and grandfathers of all the *brahmins* of the village of Paithan came to his house to eat. What a miracle! When I saw my own ancestors in Pitruloka, I became convinced that this story was not fabricated. Pitruloka really exists.

In meditation I had new experiences every day and visited many worlds. As my mind became stabilized in the Blue Pearl, Witness-consciousness would come to me. This kind of meditation can be called *samadhi*. In it one remains fully conscious. The movement of the breath becomes very soft and slow, but it does not cease as in full *kumbhaka*. This is the *samadhi* of the Siddha Path, where Witness-consciousness remains fully active. It is not an unknowing, blank *samadhi* where there is no awareness. The realm of Consciousness is that of knowledge, so the Witness-consciousness should therefore be present in true *samadhi*.

Throughout my meditation, I floated in a divine ecstasy. When it stopped, I would become conscious of the world outside me. I would relax my posture and move my arms and legs. I would go for a stroll. Whenever I sat for meditation, I would first bow to the four directions considering them to be forms of the Guru and of Parashakti. Before sitting down I would always see the place where I sat for meditation as the seat of the Guru and of the Shakti; I did not think of it just as a mat and a velvet cloth. I would see Chiti pervading above, below, everywhere. I would bow inwardly to all beings and then sit down. In the same way, when I got up from meditation, I would touch my seat and bow to it.

When I went outside after meditation that day, I could still feel the waves of love which had been coursing through all the 72,000 *nadis* during meditation. I felt completely drunk. Every cell of my blood was charged with these swirling, tossing, vibrant, ecstatic waves. I felt that I was going mad with love—not mad as I had been before; this time it was a madness of love. These waves of love that rushed through my body seemed to be telling me that I had been blessed by Parashakti.

Every day I went on meditating like this. I meditated in the morning, in the afternoon, in the evening. One of Tukaram's songs comes to mind: *tukā mhane dina rajanī hāchi dhandā*—"Tukaram says, day and night, this was my occupation." A businessman, an officer, or an employee follows a daily routine. In the morning he gets up and bathes, has breakfast, takes his lunch with him to the office, works in the office, shuts the office after work is over, and goes home. If anyone were to ask him, "What do you do?" he would say, "The same thing I do every day—come and go, eat and drink, sleep at night." And so it was with Swami Muktananda. Meditation in the morning and the evening, and when meditation was finished, work in the garden, sprinkling water. Meditation again at night, and then sleep.

Nineteen

The World of Sounds

I now arrived at a new stage in meditation called Nadaloka. There are many kinds of *nada,* resembling such things as the beating of the waves of the sea, the roll of thunder, the rippling of a stream, the rattle of a speeding train, the sound of an airplane in the distance, and the crackle of a funeral pyre. I started to hear many different sounds of this kind; sometimes I heard many voices chanting the divine name, sometimes the sounds of the *mridang* and kettledrum, sometimes the solemn and sacred sound of the conch, sometimes the mighty peals of huge bells suggesting the chanting of *Om,* sometimes the sweet singing of the *veena* and other string instruments. I also heard the sounds of honey bees, bumble bees, and other insects, the calling of the peacock in the jungle at dawn, and the cries of the cuckoo and other birds. I heard the music that I had heard before in Indraloka and other worlds. Then there were various indistinct sounds in the space within the heart. I heard one after the other—the grades of *nada: chin-chin, chinchina,* the bell, the conch, the *veena,* the cymbals, the flute, the *mridang,* the kettledrum, and thunder. In this way, I heard the ten divine sounds one after another. I became immersed in the new ecstasy that came with these sounds. Because of them I sometimes could not sleep for a whole fortnight. It seemed that sleep and *nada* were actually opposed, and I decided that sleep must have gone away sulking. However, I was not worried and my mind was not annoyed because I could not sleep. Usually when one cannot sleep for some reason, the mind is badly affected or the body suffers, but nothing of the kind happened to me. I was as energetic and happy as before, in spite of being without sleep. I felt no need for it, and I also ate less. My body began to look quite thin.

At the stage when he hears the *nada,* the yogi discovers an ability to dance. I would sometimes go at night to the top of a hill and dance for hours on end. What a wonderful divine feeling it was! I was the only one to see myself dancing. I did not show it to anyone else because it would have embarrassed me. Therefore, I danced secretly. With these graceful movements, my appetite increased a little, and my limbs felt lighter. I wondered how boys and girls and men and women of good families could shamelessly dance together in public. I wonder if perhaps I lack something because I still feel so shy. I enjoyed the *nadas,* and I also examined them very carefully. *Sadhakas* usually think that *nada* arises in the left or right ear, but actually it does not arise from the ear at all, but from the upper spaces of the *sahasrara;* it is from there that this rapturous sound arises and can be heard in either ear. I felt a sublime and divine vibration in the *akasha* within my head. My power of recollection became so strong that I could clearly re-member everyone who had ever come for my *darshan* and exactly what they had brought. I thought that if students could find the ability to retain things like this, they would not always be having to write and take notes. I remembered a line of Jnaneshwar who knew all there was to know about the Kundalini: *hechi ātmaprabhā nitya navī*—"This light of the soul is always new." And Muktananda says: *dhyāna-prabhā*—"The light of meditation is always new." I cannot tell how many new experiences I had. Though I meditated every day, my mind was never dull, and my *sadhana* never slackened. Instead, I applied my-self with growing effort and growing earnestness. Just as a man begins to run when he nears his destination, so my meditation speeded up. Every day I heard the sound of many, many *nadas.* There would often be the sweet tones of the flute. What a divine attraction that music holds! I once heard some poetry about the attraction of the flute. A *gopi* says: "O Lord, stop playing Your flute! For when You play Your flute I am not good for anything! I forget my children. I can't make myself go home. Lord, I have to go home. Listen! Please stop Your flute just for a moment. Your flute is so enchanting and so sweet that my face and my legs won't turn toward home. O, Bewitcher of the mind! Please stop playing Your flute. I have to go and feed my children. I have to give my husband his meal. His mother and father must be waiting for me. Have mercy, stop playing Your flute." So the *gopi* humbly prays to the Lord.

My dear Siddha students, when I heard the sounds of the flute in the *sahasrara,* I lost consciousness even of Tandraloka. I did not know where the inner Witness had gone. I had no idea where I was going or what was happening as I listened to the sweet music of the flute. It is not in the least surprising that the *gopis* got into such a condition when they actually heard the flute of the supremely blissful Lord Sri Krishna. There cannot be the smallest doubt about this. Those *gopis* who heard the sound of a real flute were rays of the sun of Krishna's love—a love that should be remembered with every sunrise. When a yogi becomes so absorbed in the flute *nada* he hears in the *sahasrara,* what must have been the condition of the *gopis?*

Sometimes I danced, sometimes I swayed, and sometimes I was drunk with love and lost in the divine *nada.* The *nada* is Parabrahman. It is the sound-body of Sri Guru Nityananda. It is a bursting forth of the throbbing vibrations of Parashakti Mahamaya Sri Kundalini. Its very name is *ādau bhagavān śabdarāśiḥ*—"God originally manifested as sound." I saw God in these sounds. They represented the later phase of my awakening Kundalini. As one keeps listening to the *nada,* the mind centers on the place from which it arises. I could observe the place from where sparks flew out of the divine light activated by the vibrations of the *nada.* All my senses were drawn toward it; even my tongue hurried toward it. During this phase, whenever I heard a certain *nada,* my body would react with a corresponding quivering that was slightly painful. Then it seemed that my whole body would fall to pieces. I was bathed in sweat. My head shook violently. It felt as if a gentle fire was burning throughout my body. Sometimes a tiny drop of nectar would drop from the upper *akasha,* or else sensations of the different tastes were released from there—salty, sour, bitter, and hot. Sometimes while I was listening to the *nada,* a nectar like milk trickled down my palate and then to the gastric fire, from where it went out into the 72,000 *nadis.* As a result of this, many subtle ailments of the body vanished. However much I worked my body, I never felt tired anymore. As I listened to these divine *nadas,* knowing them to be *shabda* Brahman, Brahman in the form of sound, I directly experienced *shabda* Brahman in the form of *nada.* As for my ever-active Kundalini, She too was overjoyed to be meeting Her husband who had come to Her as the *nada.* The ripples of Her delight spread right through my body. Muktananda began to dance. As the currents of the *nada* spread through his body, his mind, too, became quick and agile.

As I listened to the Lord's flute, I developed insight into many mysterious things. I heard the *nada* for longer and longer periods, and even during my everyday activities—while I was coming and going, sleeping and eating—I heard it. When I got angry, I heard it still more. The more I listened to the flute, the richer my own voice became. I benefited from the various qualities of the different *nadas* that I heard. When I heard the sound of the kettledrum, I acquired clairvoyance and could see things far away. Sometimes I would be sitting in my room and would see what was happening in another room. And it would sometimes happen that I would enter a room just when someone was doing something in secret, as if I had been called there. However, I would simply say that such and such a person had called me. I listened to the kettledrum *nada* and absorbed its virtues. My meditation progressed each day like the waxing moon.

After the *nada* of the kettledrum, I heard the final *nada,* which is called *meghanada,* the sound of thunder. It is a most divine *nada,* the king of *nada,* the celestial cow which fulfills the wishes of yogis. When it is heard, the upper space trembles. For a few days the *sadhaka* is not himself because of this continuous thundering, for this is the *nada* that leads to *samadhi,* the goal of yoga. From within this *nada,* the yogi hears the chanting of *Om.* Then he learns that *Om* is self-begotten. It is not created by sages like the various mantras of different sects. No abbot has composed it. It is self-existent. It arises by itself out of the upper spaces of the *sahasrara.* It is born of itself; it is not caused by anything else. When this *nada* comes, the yogi falls into a tremendous ecstasy. Sometimes I would forget my rule and talk to people about it. They would listen affectionately and then, to feel important, would tell other people that Swami Muktananda had heard this *nada* or that *nada.* They told Nityananda Baba also. Then, the next time I went for *darshan,* he was very angry and said, "What a fool ... talking about these things . . . revealing such secrets . . . a yogi loses what he has attained . . . suffers." Whenever he spoke like this, my *sadhana* would be held back for a few days. As I have already said many times, in Siddha Vidya: *gurukripā hi kevalam gurorājnā hi kevalam*—"Only the Guru's grace; only the Guru's command." When the Guru is displeased, it impedes *sadhana* and delays the attaining of perfection.

Every day my meditation progressed. Its only goal was the Blue Pearl. My meditation had passed through the different bodies, through the red aura to the white flame, the white flame to the black light, and now the black light to the Blue Pearl, which was surrounded by a golden halo mingled with saffron. Its luster increased every day. The more I meditated, the more brilliant it became; each day it was more luminous than the day before. But despite its ever-growing brilliance, my ever-growing ecstasy, and my ever-growing zeal, I realized in my heart that there was still something lacking, something yet to come on my way to perfection. My heart had not yet told me that I had attained perfection. Although I felt peaceful and contented, I felt there was still something left.

I now want to present a truth to a follower of meditation so that he may have firm faith and believe with all his being in the power of the Chiti Shakti and the real presence of Gurudev within the body. He should think that just as his nose, ears, eyes, tongue, and mouth exist, so does his Sri Gurudev exist within him and throughout him. Dear Siddha students! Think this over very carefully. Have a deep and genuine faith in the Guru and the divine power of grace. Just think a little. When a doctor gives an injection in any one place in your body, you can feel it spreading through the whole body. You have probably had an injection that heated up the blood in your whole body or taken a doctor's pill which rid your body of a sickness. How much virtue and power it must have to spread through every vein and particle of your body and so expel sickness from it! You have experienced this for yourself. The Sadguru himself enters you in exactly the same way—whether you are directly aware of it or not—when he initiates you through sight, word, thought, through his company, or by touching any part of the body, bringing with him the Parashakti who plays in supreme bliss and who destroys the ignorance that causes all your afflictions. The Guru becomes incarnate within you from head to toe as your seven bodily components, your ten senses, your five sheaths. So it is not at all difficult for you to receive guidance from within and attain realization. But if you turn away from the wisdom of such a Guru, from his love, from faith in him and obedience to him, he will turn away from you. He is incarnate inside you in the form of *kriyas*. So, when he lives within you, it is no miracle that he can teach you things from within. What Muktananda says is true: the Guru is completely yours in every sense, but you have not become completely his. He is not at all far from you; it is you who are far from him. This is why you do not have new realizations every day.

I had really firm faith in my Guru. Wherever I went, I always had to carry his photograph. If I went for a walk, I had his photograph with me. When I sat down to eat, I had his photograph with me. I took his photograph with me when I went to sleep. I even kept it in my bathroom—I didn't care what people said.

In the inner light, which is of the form of Sri Gurudev, the Sarvajnaloka that I described earlier, I now received a message: "O, Muktananda, though you have achieved *jivanmukti* from the vision of the Blue Pearl and have experienced transcendental bliss, you have still to achieve complete perfection. What you have is not yet divine realization. For that you must enter the Blue Pearl." This was a message from the Goddess Chiti within me. I took it as Her true command and meditated even more. The more I meditated, the longer the Blue Pearl would stand steadily before me, and the longer it stayed, the more its brightness increased. As long as it was there, it would display ever new ways and miracles. Infinite feelings began to well up within me, such as: Is it just blue or is it Neelakantha, Shiva with a blue throat? Is it just blue or is it a blue Sri Nityananda? It is just blue or is it Neeleshwari, the Blue Goddess, Bhavani Uma Shakti Kundalini? The Blue Pearl came closer and closer. The more it grew, the more it shone, and the more Muktananda grew, the more he changed, the more he opened, the more he expanded and realized what Muktananda really was. Whatever was happening to the Blue Pearl was happening to Muktananda. My faith in the Blue Pearl became still stronger, and just as you think in relation to different parts of the body—"they are mine" and "that is me"—so I came to think of the Blue Pearl.

Twenty

The Vision of the Blue Person

O my dear Siddha students. Now something new happened. Listen to this with love, and don't ever forget what I am telling you. One day I was sitting in joyful meditation. As soon as I sat down, I started the great worship of Sadguru Nityananda, who is one with the Goddess Kundalini Shakti. "O Gurudev, you are on my east, you are on my west, you are to my north, you are to my south. O Sadguru, you are above me, you are below me. O Dear Sri Guru, you are in my eyes, you are in my ears, you are in my nose, you are in my mouth. O Sadgurunath, giver of grace! You are in my throat, you are in my arms, you are in my chest, you are in my back, you are in my stomach. O mother Guru! O father Guru! You are in my thighs, you are in my legs, you are in my feet. O my Baba! You are in me, I am in you. And you are in any difference there may be between my form and yours." I invoked my Guru in this way, and my meditation began with the red aura glittering before me. Then the white flame, the black light, and the Blue Pearl followed one after the other. My heart was filled with joy. Megharaja, lord of the clouds and friend of yogis, was thundering inside the *sahasrara*. Then a great miracle happened. I should not talk about it, but Sri Guru is urging me to do so. I do not have the strength to write about this miracle. My hand does not move. My fingers have stopped working. My eyes will not open. Only my tongue is moving. Perhaps Nityananda has come and forcibly taken possession of it. Since I do not have the right to speak, it is Bhagavan Nityananda who is speaking. My dear friend Yande is doing the writing. He has surrendered himself to Baba Nityananda, which is why he is writing.

The wonderfully radiant Blue Pearl, with its countless different rays shining from within, came closer to me and began to grow. It assumed the shape of an egg and continued to grow into a human shape. I could see it growing with my own eyes and was lost in utmost amazement. The egg grew and grew until it had assumed the shape of a man. Suddenly divine radiance burst forth from it. For a moment I lost consciousness. What had happened to Tandraloka? Where had Sarvajnaloka gone? And what had become of the intuitive intelligence by which I had understood everything so far? Muktananda forgot himself for a few moments. Because he did not exist, everything else also disappeared. If there is no one to see, there is nothing seen. If there is no one to listen, there is no sound. If there is no one to smell, there is no smell. For a moment I was not conscious of anything. However, my state of meditation was still just as it had been. I was sitting firmly in the lotus posture, facing north. Then, I again saw a shining human form in place of the oval. As it shone, Muktananda came back to himself. Muktananda's Tandraloka returned. Intuitive intelligence came back and also Muktananda's extraordinary memory, which was always watching over and reporting his inner states.

The egg-shaped Blue Pearl stood before me in the form of a man. Its brightness lessened. I saw within it a Blue Person. What a beautiful form he had! His blueness shone and scintillated. His body was not the product of human fluids derived from the seven elements, but of the blue rays of pure Consciousness, which Tukaram Maharaj called *chinmay anjan*—"the lotion of Consciousness that grants divine vision." His body was composed of infinite rays of Consciousness. He was a mass of Consciousness, the essence of Muktananda's inner life, the real form of Nityananda. He was the true form of my Mother, the playful, divine Kundalini. He stood before me, shimmering and resplendent in His divinity.

What a beautiful body He had! What beautiful eyes! What a fine straight nose! What attractive ears and earrings, and what beautiful hair! How fine His head! He had no beard. He wore on His head a crown set with the nine jewels. These were not inert material creations of this earth, but were composed of pure Consciousness. What beautiful long hands, slender fingers and nails He had—all so blue. The clothes He wore were soft and fine. How long and shapely His legs, and how well formed His toes. His whole body was exquisitely beautiful. I kept gazing at Him, from head to toe, from toe to head, my eyes wide in amazement.

He came toward me, making a soft humming sound, and made some kind of gesture. "Say something," He said. What could I say? I was completely absorbed in just looking at Him. He walked right around me and stood still. Then, looking at me, He made a sign with His eyes. Then He said, "I see everything from everywhere. I see with My eyes. I see with My nose. I have eyes everywhere." He lifted up a foot a little and said, "I see with this foot, too. I can see everywhere. I have tongues everywhere. I speak not just with My tongue, but also with My hand, and with My foot. I have ears everywhere. I can hear with every part of My body." Thus He spoke, and I listened to Him. "I move with My feet, and also with My head. I can move any way I like. I move as far as I want in an instant. I walk without feet and catch without hands. I speak without a tongue, and I see without eyes. While I am far, far away, I am very near. I become the body in all bodies, and yet I am different from the body." Then He said a little more, which was heard by Nityananda and cannot be written here. Then He added, "This very way is the path of the Siddhas, the true way." He lifted His hand, and made a gesture of blessing. I was utterly amazed. As I watched, the blue egg, which had grown to a height of six feet, now began to shrink. It became smaller and smaller until it was once more Neeleshwari. It became my Blue Light, the Blue Pearl.

I was completely amazed. Filled with great bliss and thinking only of the grace of Sri Gurudev Bhagavan Nityananda and of the divine Sri Chiti Kundalini, I passed into Tandraloka. I realized that this was the *neela purusha*, the Blue Person, who grants the realization of God with Form. He is also called the supreme unmanifest Being, by whose blessing one proceeds to the realization of the ultimate Truth. After blessing me, this Being returned into the Blue Pearl from which He had emerged; and then my meditation ceased.

How marvelous are the countless visions in the world of meditation! How great is man's worthiness! How magnificant is the Blue Pearl! How bountiful is Dhyaneshwara, the lord of meditation!

How glorious is man, how magnificent he is! O Muktananda! You are great. You are infinite. You are extraordinary. I was completely overcome with joy, giving thanks for my human birth and recalling what I had seen. Now the conviction "I am the Self," became firmly established. I believed completely in *So'ham hamsah,* "He is I, I am He"— "You are God, God is in you." I began to experience the full realization of this truth.

I was convinced that this was the divine Being who had been described in the *Gita* (13:13-14):

> *sarvatah pāṇipādaṁ tat sarvato 'kshiśiromukham*
> *sarvatah śrutimalloke sarvamāvratya tiṣthati*

He has hands and feet everywhere. He has eyes, heads, and faces on all sides. He has ears everywhere. He knows all and exists pervading all.

> *sarvendriyaguṇābhāsaṁ sarvendriyavivarjitam*
> *asaktaṁ sarvabhruchchaiva nirguṇaṁ guṇabhoktr cha*

He has all the qualities of the senses and yet is without any of the qualities of the senses, unattached and yet supporting all, free from the three attributes of manifestation and yet enjoying them.

He dwells in the *sahasrara* and appears in subtle form in the powers of all the sense organs. He can be experienced by the senses and yet is far beyond them and without them. While in the body, He says, "I am Muktananda, I am, I am," yet He is unattached to it. He is the nourisher of all. He is the sustainer of every cell within the 72,000 *nadis,* the One who nourishes by giving vitality to the vital fluids and richness to the blood. He is beyond the three *gunas,* and yet, even though He has none of the *gunas,* He dwells within the *sahasrara* and experiences all *gunas.* If someone gives food, He eats it; if someone gives flowers, He accepts them; if someone gives clothes, He wears them; if someone bows He accepts that too. The person giving all these things thinks, "I am giving them to Baba," but it is He who accepts them:

> *bahirantashcha bhūtānāmacharaṁ charameva cha*
> *sūkshmatvāttadavijneyaṁ dūrasthaṁ chāntike cha tat*
>
> (*Gita* 13:15)

That is without and within all beings, the unmoving and also the moving, unknowable because of its subtlety, and near and far away.

He pervades the outer and inner aspects of the movable and immovable creation—men and demons, birds and animals, insects and germs—but because He does so in His subtle form, He is not understood. People think that He lives far away, but He lives very close to you, in the middle of the *sahasrara.* This supreme Being appears to be different in different people, races, actions, names, forms, countries, and times, but He is undifferentiated. He lives as human being in a human being, as bird in a bird, as cow in a cow, as horse in a horse, as man in a man, and as woman in a woman. What else can I say? He becomes all things and is yet unique. He gives His strength to all created things. Like a mother He protects and sustains them and then gathers them all into Himself. He is the supreme light of all lights; all lights take their brightness from Him. There is no darkness about Him. He knows everything about everything. If this were not so, how could Muktananda have recognized the Blue Person? What I had seen was the Blue Pearl; it was Shiva, the Blue Lord; it was blue Nityananda, who is the highest object of knowledge, who is the gift of Kundalini's grace received in the highest states of meditation, who is apprehended only with the knowledge acquired in Sarvajnaloka, and who dwells in His total fullness in the heart and in the *sahasrara.* O seekers! He is within your Blue Pearl, but do not think that you have become perfect just because you have seen the Blue Pearl. That supreme unmanifest Being is extremely secret to *sadhakas;* He is the goal of the Siddha Path. This is not something that can ever be expressed in speech or writing, even at the end of time. It is only by His grace that divine realization will come. Siddha students will understand how this matter, which should not be written, has been written. I am compelled to speak, and dear Yande is taking it down.

But even with all this, my contentment was still incomplete. There was still something left. The stage my meditation had reached was very divine. The Blue Person I had seen is also known as the Sphere of unmanifest Light. Yogis see Him, who contains the entire world within Himself, within the Blue Pearl in meditation. I was now meditating on Him and constantly remembering Him. He had settled in the land of my mind and had taken a form. I meditated constantly and always saw the sweet, radiant Blue Pearl in its infinite variations. Its luster was more dazzling at each moment, and my enjoyment was forever growing. I was meditating in the *sahasrara* and was also hearing the divine *nada* of thunder. As I listened to this thundering, my meditation became so joyful that the desires which remained in my mind were smashed by the thunder and just disappeared. As I listened to this sound for a while I experienced complete union with the taintless Parabrahman.

The *sadhaka* should never forget that Mahashakti Kundalini, who is the treasure house of inner knowledge and dwells in the *muladhara,* when awakened by the grace of the Guru, will secure what he doesn't already possess and preserve what he does possess. The more the *sadhaka* takes refuge in the Kundalini and the Guru, the more they will stand before him for his protection. He must constantly remember to take his sole refuge in the Guru and the Shakti. When I call this Mahashakti the divine power of grace, the Siddha student should understand that it is Kundalini, it is the Guru, it is God. Just as a needle on touching a piece of cloth pierces and passes right through it, so the Mahashakti Kundalini rises from the *muladhara,* at the base of the spine, and goes up the *sushumna,* the central channel, to the *brahma-randhra,* the spiritual center in the crown of the head, piercing the *chakras* on Her way. The *sadhaka* feels the touch of the Kundalini in his body. When She is awakened and spreads through the 72,000 *nadis,* the *sadhaka* becomes aware of Her soft, tender, joyous, divine touch. Sometimes Her touch is harsh, and then the whole body feels as if it is on fire. Whether Her touch is soft or hard depends on the nature of the aspirant. But either way, it is the touch of God.

When the mind is turned upward into the *sahasrara* and becomes stable in meditation there, the sound of thunder is heard and the tongue turns up against the soft palate. Then the aspirant starts to taste a divine savor. Sometimes when the tongue is in this position, one can taste the cool nectar of the moon, and the Siddha student is full of delight and amazement. He meditates with even more enthusiasm so that he can drink more and more of the nectar. There can also be tastes of butter, milk, *ghee,* buttermilk, honey, and other things. These come when the *sadhaka's* mind becomes absorbed in the *ajna chakra,* and he sees his Self as the wickless flame in the space between the eyebrows. When he tastes these different nectars, many inner sicknesses are dispelled. When he meditates more and his *prana* becomes stabilized in this place, the aspirant experiences divine fragrances. One can reach a very high state when one smells these. I had many, many experiences like these and my meditation steadily progresssed.

After my vision of the Blue Person, my meditation became stabilized in the upper space of the *sahasrara,* where I saw a celestial radiance like a mist, and in the midst of this radiance, the Blue Pearl. This brightness increased day by day. It is always found around the Blue Pearl, and it is said that the radiance of the firmament within the *sahasrara* comes from the splendor of the Blue Pearl. I meditated on it every day, and each day there arose the awareness, "I am the Self." Sometimes I would also see the Blue Pearl moving in and out of the *sahasrara* for short periods. If you ever have a vision of the coming of a great saint, you should understand that it is all happening through the agency of the Blue Pearl.

Twenty-one
Fear of Death

Another amazing thing now happened to me in meditation. There came a stage when my eyes would roll upward during my meditation, and my eyelids would also be drawn up. My pupils would be focused on the Blue Pearl in the middle of the *sahasrara*. My neck would be stretched a little upward. I have already described the Sphere of unmanifest Light found in the *sahasrara*. One day it opened up and its light was released, and the brilliance of not one or two thousand, but millions of suns blazed all around. The light was so fierce that I could not stand it, and my courage broke down. I no longer had the power to stop my meditation. I could not get up from where I was sitting. My posture was not under my control, nor could I open or shut my eyes at will. That brilliance had drawn me toward itself, and as I gazed at it, I lost consciousness. When I recovered myself a little, I began to cry, "O Goddess, O Sadgurunath, save me!" because I was afraid of dying. My *prana* had stopped moving; my mind was not working. I felt that my *prana* was passing out of my body. "O Lord, O Sadguru," I cried, *"Om, Om,"* and then I lost all control over my body. Just as a dying man opens his mouth, spreads his arms, and makes a strange sound, so I fell down making this sort of noise. As I fell, I urinated involuntarily, which made me feel that I had completely lost consciousness.

I lay in this unknown state of unconsciousness for about an hour or an hour and a half, and then, as a man rises from sleep, I got up and laughed to myself, saying, "I just died, but now I'm alive again." I got up feeling very much at peace, very happy, and very full of love. I realized that I had experienced death when I saw the unmanifest divine radiance as bright as millions of suns. I had been very frightened, but from this experience I now understood death. I realized that death is nothing but this condition. Once I had seen that Sphere of unmanifest Light I lost all fear. This is the state of liberation from individual existence. Since then my courage has increased a great deal, and I no longer know any fear. I am not afraid of anything. I never think about what is going to happen. I never worry about what somebody will do. The place of fear within me has been destroyed. I have attained total fearlessness.

Now the awareness of the Self began to rise within me spontaneously. Formerly the feeling *deho 'ham*—"I am the body," had always throbbed within me; but now it had all changed, and it was the feeling *shivo 'ham* —"I am Shiva," that pulsated within of its own accord. The rapture of bliss was steadily increasing. All those memories of the form of the supreme Blue Being, of His blessing, of His living within me, of my identification with Him, of "I am He"—all rang within me. I began to sway in the rapture of the sound of the *nada*, in the intensity of the love that spread through every part of my body, and in the memory of my fear of being destroyed by that divine Sphere of unmanifest light. There came more and deeper meditation, more profound experiences of the Self. Yet even then something inside me said that there was still further to go. I began to feel a lack of something, but there was nothing I could do about it. There was only one way to fill this lack: complete and unconditional surrender to the inner Shakti, who was Sri Gurudev. I went on meditating, and every day I saw that divine, radiant Sphere and the Blue Pearl inside it and heard the *nada* of the thunder. That was the state of my meditation.

Sometimes I would have fleeting visions of the all-knowing Blue Being, as quick as flashes of lightning. My meditation became deeper. Every day my conviction became stronger: "He is truly my inner Self, whose light is spread throughout the entire universe." Although I could not see it directly, I saw my inner Self as the Blue Person. Through the gift of Bhagavan Sri Nityananda's grace, I was gaining the realization that the Blue One was my own Self, the One who lives within all, pervades the entire universe and sets it in motion, who is one-without-a-second, nondual and undifferentiated, and yet is always at play, becoming many from one and one from many. He is Sri Krishna, the eternal Blue of Consciousness, the beloved life-breath of the *gopis*, and the Self of yogis. This inner, eternal Blue of Consciousness is the *So'ham Brahma*—"I am He, the Absolute," of *jnanis*. This Blue is the adorable one chose by *bhaktas*, who fills them with the nectar of love. This eternal Blue of Consciousness is Muktananda Swami's own beloved deity, Sri Guru Nityananda. This eternal Blue of Consciousness is the Siddha students' divine power of grace. If this is not realized, we cannot understand that the universe appears within God, the Absolute. But with the knowledge given to us by Parashakti Kundalini as She unfolds and grows within us, we can see the universe at play in the form of the Godhead.

I began to see that He, through whose grace *maya* becomes known as the manifestation of the Lord, is my Self appearing as the Blue Pearl. I began to see that the Blue One, whose light spreads through the whole world, the One from whom I received knowledge, who is the pure transcendent Witness of all, the unchanging Being, the unchanging Truth, is my inner Self. I became firmly established in the inner knowledge that just as the sun is visible and yet cannot be seen by the blind, in the same way, even though the Blue of Consciousness, the Witness of all, is apparent, it cannot be seen without the grace of the Guru. But a cloud cannot obscure the sun forever. He who reveals Himself for a moment and hides Himself for a moment, yet is revealed even when hidden, is my Self. I began to believe that He who takes care of my yogic *sadhana*, who was known to our ancestors, and who will be known to those who are to come, by whose grace our attachment to the world disappears, was my being, my consciousness, and my bliss. A firm and steadfast belief arose within me that that Blue One—who makes light shine, and who shines also in inert matter, without knowledge of whom all knowledge is incomplete, and with whose knowledge all things are easily known—was the form of the grace of Sri Guru Nityananda. And yet, while these convictions were becoming stronger, I had a subtle feeling that there was still a little more to go. The great Kundalini continually deepened my meditation and my knowledge of the Absolute.

Twenty-three

The Dawn of Knowledge

Through my reflections after meditation, I came to understand the goal of the Vedantins. In my meditation, the knowledge came by itself of that supreme Truth that is realized by the Vedantins through the Witness-consciousness, when the mind is in absolute stillness. I understood that Truth in which the most subtle intellect loses itself while probing it. The merging of the intellect into that Truth is the attainment of Vedanta. While man is awake, That which perceives the whole external world as *idam,* "this," as object, and yet remains aloof from and transcends the waking state; That which, when man is asleep and dreaming, does not sleep but remains awake, and with neither the mind nor the senses perceives the whole dream universe as "this,"; and when man is in the black depths of dreamless sleep where nothing is seen, That which remains as the illuminator and perceives this state of nothingness—I began to understand That as the unchanging Self, the supreme goal of meditation. The knowledge that the witnessing Self, which sits in the eyes and makes us see forms, which lives in the ears and conveys the import of words to the other senses, which activates the movement of breathing in and out, and yet remains steady and unchanging in the midst of this movement, is the goal of Vedanta, arose spontaneously from within. Under the dominion of ignorance man says, "I ate, I drank, I took, I gave," but the One who experiences all these things is the unmoving Witness, the inner Self—and that is God. Having realized this, I would wonder, when different types of people came to me crying and complaining, whether they were speaking the truth or telling lies. And the feeling would arise in me that the inner Self within me was also in them. I came to see that just as a painter might paint many pictures on one canvas with just one color, one brush, and one concept, in the same way, there is One in this universe, despite all the different forms and colors that may be seen. I came to see, in other words, that in all differences there is identity.

In this way, I was gaining more and more knowledge, but I did not let my meditation lose its edge or relax my *sadhana*. As I meditated, my vision became steadily fixed on the *sahasrara* and the pupils of my eyes were drawn toward it. And then something new happened, something that is beyond words. I do not know how I am still talking about it. Now my dear Professor Jain is writing it down. The inevitable does come to pass. It is the will of God that prevails. It is true that "Rama, the Lord, makes everyone dance!"

Twenty-four
Final Realization

My meditation was approaching its fulfillment. The end of my *sadhana,* the completion of my spiritual journey, the complete satisfaction of my Self, was coming near. The time had come for my Gurudev's command to be fulfilled. I was to reach the summit of man's fortune, which is divine realization. Once the vehicle of a spiritual traveler's *sadhana* has reached this point, it stops there forever. There, you may see nothing and hear nothing, but at the same time all is seen and heard, for inside you is the spontaneous conviction that you have attained everything. When an aspirant has reached there, he sits in bliss, sleeps in bliss, walks in bliss, comes and goes in bliss. He lives in an ashram in bliss, he eats in bliss; his behavior and actions are blissful. He experiences directly, "Now I have crossed the ocean of worldly existence." By virtue of this realization he is never agitated. No matter what he is doing, his heart is as calm as the ocean. All the afflictions of the mind melt away, and it becomes transmuted into Chiti. From inside comes the voice, "I am that which is dear to all, the Self of all, I am, I am." Now once again I saw Neeleshvara, the Blue Lord, whose nature is Satchidananda—Being, Consciousness, and Bliss. Seeing Him, the *sadhaka* enjoys happiness free from duality. He acquires supreme knowledge free from doubts, and knowledge of the identity of all things.

My very own, my dear Siddha students. My meditation was again as it had been earlier. From within, Bhagavan Nityananda seemed to shake me, and then the rays of the red aura lit up the 72,000 *nadis* and all the particles of blood. Immediately afterward the white flame stood before me, followed by her support, the black light, and finally my beloved Blue Pearl, the great ground of all. With the Blue Pearl my meditation immediately became more intense. My gaze turned upward. The Blue *bindu* of my two eyes became so powerful that it drew out the Blue Person hidden within the *brahmarandhra* in the middle of the upper *sahasrara* and placed Him before me. As I gazed at the tiny Blue Pearl, I saw it expand, spreading its radiance in all directions so that the whole sky and earth were illuminated by it. It was now no longer a Pearl but had become shining, blazing, infinite Light; the Light which the writers of the scriptures and those who have realized the Truth have called the divine Light of Chiti. The Light pervaded everywhere in the form of the universe. I saw the earth being born and expanding from the Light of Consciousness, just as one can see smoke rising from a fire. I could actually see the world within this conscious Light, and the Light within the world, like threads in a piece of cloth, and cloth in the threads. Just as a seed becomes a tree, with branches, leaves, flowers, and fruit, so within Her own being Chiti becomes animals, birds, germs, insects, gods, demons, men, and women. I could see this radiance of Consciousness, resplendent and utterly beautiful, silently pulsing as supreme ecstasy within me, outside me, above me, below me. I was meditating even though my eyes were open. Just as a man who is completely submerged in water can look around and say, "I am in the midst of water, I am surrounded on all sides by water; there is nothing else," so was I completely surrounded by the Light of Consciousness. In this condition the phenomenal world vanished and I saw only pure radiance. Just as one can see the infinite rays of the sun shimmering in all directions, so the Blue Light was sending out countless rays of divine radiance all about it.

I was no longer aware of the world around me. I was deep in divine feeling. And then, in the midst of the spreading blue rays, I saw Sri Gurudev, his hand raised in blessing. I saw my adored, my deity, Sri Nityananda. I looked again, and, instead, Lord Parashiva with his trident was standing there. He was so beautiful, so charming. He was made solely of blue light. Hands, feet, nails, head, hair were all pure blueness. As I watched, He changed, as Nityananda had changed, and now I could see Muktananda as I had seen him once before when I had had the vision of my own form. He too was within the Blue Light of Consciousness; his body, his shawl, his rosary of *rudraksha* seeds were all of the same blue. Then there was Shiva again, and after Shiva, Nityananda within the Blue. The Blue Light was still the same, with the sparkling luster of its rays and its wonderful blue color. How beautiful it was! Nityananda was standing in the midst of the shimmering radiance of pure Consciousness and then, as ice melts into water, as camphor evaporates into air, he merged into it. There was now just a mass of shining radiant Light with no name and form. Then all the rays bursting forth from the Blue Light contracted and returned into the Blue Pearl. The Blue Pearl was once again the size of a tiny lentil seed. The Pearl went to the place from where it had come, merging into the *sahasrara*. Merging into the *sahasrara*, Muktananda lost his consciousness, memory, distinctions of inner and outer, and the awareness of himself. Here I have not revealed a supreme secret because Gurudev does not command me to do so, God does not wish it, and the Siddhas do not instruct me to write it.

Now I went into inner *samadhi* and some time passed in this way. Then as Witness-consciousness began to return, the Blue Light appeared, which Shankaracharya describes as *sat chinmaya neelima,* the eternal Blue of Consciousness. My meditation became focused on it. I began to experience that I was entering into the center of the *sahasrara* and the Blue Pearl, the support of all. As I passed inside the Blue Pearl, I once again saw the universe spreading out in all directions. I looked around everywhere and saw in all men and women—young and old, high and low, in each and every one—that same Blue Pearl that I had seen in myself. I saw that this was the inner Self within everyone's *sahasrara,* and with this full realization my meditation stopped, and I returned to normal body-consciousness. I still saw the Blue Pearl with my inner mind. It drew my attention toward itself, and as I looked at it, I attained peace and equanimity. My meditation continued like this every day.

I still meditate now, but I have a deep certainty that there is nothing more for me to see. When I meditate, the certainty that I have attained full realization fills me completely. I say this because of the three kinds of visions that I saw within the Blue Pearl and because in the outer world I still see that same Light of Consciousness, whose subtle, tranquil blue rays I had seen spreading everywhere after the three visions. It has never gone away. When I shut my eyes, I still see it shimmering and shining, softer than soft, more tender than tender, finer than fine. When the eyes are open, I see the blue rays all around. Whenever I see anyone, I see first the Blue Light and then the person. Whenever I see anything, I see first the beautiful subtle rays of Consciousness, and then the thing itself. Wherever my mind happens to turn, I see the world in the midst of this shining mass of Light. The way I see things, whether large or small, demonstrates the truth of the verses of Tukaram, which I have quoted before: "My eyes have been bathed with the lotion of the Blue Light, and I have been granted divine vision."

Twenty-five

The Play of Consciousness

Even now when I meditate, as soon as I am absorbed in meditation, I see the mass of the blue rays of the Light of Consciousness and within that the Blue Pearl. I see this soft, gleaming Consciousness pulsating so delicately and shining in all my states. Whether I am eating or drinking or bathing it comes and stands before my eyes. Even when I am sleeping it is there. Now my vision is neither dual nor nondual, because that radiance is in both. There is no longer any demarcation between space, time, and substance. The Blue Light, subtly spreading everywhere, pervades my own being as it does the whole universe. I even see what is invisible. Just as with the lotion of mantras one can see an invisible and secret treasure, so the blue lotion, applied to my eyes by the grace of Sri Gurudev and the blessing of the divine Kundalini, has granted me divine realization, so that I can see that which is too subtle to be seen. Now I really know that my Self pervades everywhere as the universe. I am completely convinced that there is no such entity as the phenomenal world, that indeed there never was such an entity. What we call the universe is nothing other than the conscious play of Chiti Shakti. I have naturally and easily understood the significance of the *sah,* "He," and *aham,* "I," which combine to form *So'ham.* That knowledge described in Vedanta as "Thou are That," whose fruit is the bliss of the Absolute, is my very own Self gently vibrating within me. To confirm this I give an aphorism from the *Pratyabhijnahridayam,* which describes the viewpoint of Shiva, the supreme Self:

śrīmatparamaśivasya punaḥ viśvottīrṇa
viśvātmaka paramānandamaya
prakāśaikaghanasya evaṁvidhameva
śivādi dharaṇyantaṁ akhilaṁ
abhedenaiva sphurati na tu vastutaḥ
anyat kiṅchit grāhyaṁ grāhakaṁ vā;
api tu śrīparamaśivabhaṭṭāraka eva itthaṁ
nānāvaichitryasahasraiḥ sphurati

This means that for Lord Parashiva, whom we also call Parameshvara and Parashakti, there is no such thing as the universe. He is true, eternal, attributeless, formless, all-pervasive, and perfect. He sees the whole universe, from Shiva to the earth—the moving and the unmoving, the manifest and the unmanifest—as supremely blissful Light, undifferentiated from Himself. There is nothing other than He; distinctions of seer and seen, subject and object, individual and universal, and matter and consciousness are not real. It is the vibrations of Lord Parashiva alone that produce the countless different forms of the universe. I see that the universe is the body of the Lord, and that Paramashiva Himself appears as the universe within His own being.

Jnaneshwar says in the last two verses of the poem that made me start writing *Chitshakti Vilas*:

tayāchā makaraṅda svarūpa teṁ śuddha brahmādikā bodha hāchī jhālā
jñānadeva mhaṇe nivṛitti prasādeṁ nijarūpa govindeṁ janīṁ pāhatāṁ

> The blissful essence of the Blue Lord which I have described here is the true nature of God. This has been the experience of all sages, from Brahma onward. My innermost form, envisioned by the favor of Sadguru Nivrittinath, is truly Govinda, the supreme Lord. I see Him everywhere.

Vedanta states that nothing exists apart from the all-pervasive Godhead, and this is true. In fact, the whole point of life is to acquire this knowledge of God, and once we have gained it, our life becomes full of nectar. This knowledge is absolutely necessary to man, and it can be gained only through Shaktipat. All the great saints have found God within themselves through the grace of the Siddhas. The experience of Jnaneshwar quoted above is completely representative of them all. The inner Self, discovered by Janaka, Sanaka, Narada, and other sages, is the very essence of that knowledge which bestows the highest bliss and which has been handed down through the ages. The supremely blissful Lord Govinda can be seen within all men. He can be seen within everyone, whether enlightened or ignorant, whether a fool or a madman, for madness and foolishness are just states of mind, whereas the Self is perfectly pure. The Being who is beyond the sixteen *kalas* dwells constantly in the center of *brahmarandhra* in the midst of a thousand petals. Above the sixteen *kalas* is a seventeenth; that is the Self. When one's vision has been completely purified, one can see the form of the Self as a blue color in the *sahasrara*. Jnaneshwar says that he is revealing this great secret truth through the grace of his Sadguru.

In reality the universe is a divine sport; it is the playful pastime of Consciousness, the blossoming of Chiti Shakti. Because of ignorance of Chiti, the world appears. When knowledge of Chiti arises, then the whole world disappears, and only Chiti is seen everywhere.

The sage Vasuguptacharya has said truly:

> *iti vā yasya saṁvittih krīḍātvenākhilaṁ jagat*
> *sa puśyansatataṁ yukto jīvanmukto na saṁśayah*

> (*Spanda Shastra*)

He who continually perceives this entire universe as a sport of the universal Consciousness is truly Self-realized beyond any doubt; he is liberated in this body.

The world in which we live is a play of Chiti Shakti, the self-luminous universal Consciousness. For a man who sees this, the world is nothing but a play of God's energy. For him there is no bondage and no liberation. There is no means, no goal, and no limitation. By the blessing of the Guru, his eye of wisdom has been opened. The veil of duality, which made him see differences, has been torn. If he has not received the Guru's grace, the divine and playful Chiti will not come and take possession of his eyes and will not allow the true nature of the universe to be revealed. With the Guru's grace She enters the Siddha student, spreads through his whole body, and completely purifies it. She makes him like Herself, and takes possession of his eyes, his heart, and his mind. The Siddha student then sees the world as the sport of Chiti Shakti. This is the true vision. This is what Vasuguptacharya declared when he said that the world is not a separate object but a game of the universal Consciousness.

By Her very nature Chiti is supremely free. She is self-luminous. She holds within Herself the threefold power of creation, sustenance, and dissolution. She is the fundamental cause of everything, and at the same time She is the means to happiness. Though She transcends space, time, and form, She becomes all three. All space, all time, and all form appear only through Her agency. Even though Chiti manifests as the world, because She is all-pervasive, ever-perfect, and ever-luminous, She is complete in Her unity and oneness.

> *deśakālākārabhedaḥ samvido na hi yujyate*
> *tasmādekaiva pūrṇāham vimarśātmā chiduchyate*

There is no difference of space, time, or form in Consciousness. Therefore, Consciousness is said to be One alone, in the form of the experience of perfect I-ness.

When Paramashiva wishes to create, Chiti expands Herself of Her own accord, accepts differentiation in Herself, and manifests through innumerable forms. In Her creative aspect, Chiti shines forth in the external world as the body of the whole universe. This is called the immanent aspect of Chiti. But though She appears as the universe, Chiti is above and beyond it, remaining self-illumined, pure, and immaculate in Her transcendent aspect. In the same way, in Her creative outgoing aspect as the conscious Self of man, She takes on from head to toe innumerable states and forms, becoming the gross, subtle, causal, and supracausal bodies; the five sheaths; the four states; the four inner instruments; the thirty-six principles of the physical body, which is composed of the five gross elements, the 72,000 *nadis,* the seven bodily components, the five senses of perception, the five organs of action and their objects, and the five forms of *prana* and their functions. She creates innumerable conditions and forms, such as happiness, suffering, fear, disease, change, childhood, youth, heaven, hell, and She Herself enters them, thus becoming the very form of the phenomenal world. But even then She never loses Her immaculate purity. Chiti plays in the external world and yet stays always the same.

In Her transcendental aspect, above and beyond the universe, She is different from the waking state and from all the good and bad actions of the body in the waking state, from dreaming and all that happens in dreams, and from deep sleep and the nothingness of deep sleep. She is in the supracausal *turiya* state and is yet beyond it. She is within every part of the universe as the never-perturbed Witness of everything in it, and yet She is different from the universe.

Within the Blue Pearl there is only the blissful, sweet, and beautiful Chiti. There is nothing other than Her, there is nothing else like Her. In Her unity, in Her role as the Witness, She is supreme Shiva, supreme Consciousness, absolutely alone. There is nothing before Her, in the middle of Her, or behind Her. In this mode She is called the transcendent supreme Shiva, the "formless, attributeless Absolute" of the Vedantins. She has two aspects: the supremely pure transcendent aspect, which is above the world, and the immanent aspect, in which, by Her own desire, She becomes the universe within Her own being.

Siddha students, here is something for you to think about. When you have received the blessings of the Guru, and you gain the real fruit and dwell for a while in the upper *sahasrara,* entirely absorbed in your own happiness, then you do not experience anything other than yourself, nor do you see anything other than yourself, nor does anything else exist. There is only you yourself. Then you enjoy your own bliss, the ecstasy of the Guru's grace within your own being. This is known as *purnahanta,* the state in which one experiences one's own completeness, the state of "I am perfect." This is the resting place of Siddha students. Here you perceive your own Self within your being. This is the true *aham* or "I."

If anyone asks what is the nature of this "I," you should say that It is Brahman, Shiva, Rama, Shakti, Kundalini, and that It is also the Siddha student. As *aham*, this "I" passes out of the transcendent state into the state of immanence, It becomes *idam*, or "this"—the object. It passes from the *turiya* state to that of deep sleep, from deep sleep to dreaming, from dreaming to wakefulness, and then from head to toe It becomes the whole body of the universe. In this, Its immanent aspect, It plays in the field of the three *gunas.* From the supreme transcendent state called *turiyatita* to the waking state, It manifests itself by its own desire. Yet even when It has become the universe It does not forget its own nature; It does not destroy its integrity or become anything else. Thus, of Its own free will and within Its own being, It creates the world.

Chiti has two aspects—the perceiver and the perceived. The whole aggregate of the outer universe, which is understood as *idam*, as "this," is the perceived; whereas the inner power which knows "this" from within, which sees things separately as "this pot," "this cloth," is the perceiver. The entire universe is the field of the perceived while the perceiver is the universal Self. The perceived universe exists in accordance with the nature of the perceiver, and is meant only for the perceiver to enjoy. Thus, the all-powerful Chiti, the performer of an infinity of marvels, becomes the universe and the universal Self as the perceiver and the perceived. Chiti is the play of the world; and the world is the play of Chitshakti.

According to Kashmir Shaivism:

> *śarīrameva ghaṭādyapi vā ye ṣaṭatriṁśattattvamayaṁ*
> *śivarūpatayā paśyanti te'pi sidhyanti*

This means that the Siddha student who sees this body as a form of Chiti made of the thirty-six constituent principles, that is, as the body of Paramashiva Himself, attains all realizations, according to the laws of the Siddha Science. Chiti is playing in both Her differentiated and undifferentiated forms. Just as the four states of man—waking, dreaming, deep sleep, and *turiya*—are his own and not different from him, so the body of the universe is Chiti's own body, and not different from Her.

All the scriptures declare this same principle: The Absolute is Satchidananda—Being, Consciousness, and Bliss. The world, which is born from the Absolute, is not different from It. All these appearances —"I," "you," "this,"—are simply His play. Identity appearing in diversity, diversity appearing in identity—all this is the Lord. This is the true principle. Just as the innumerable drops, foam, bubbles, and waves of the ocean are in no way different from the ocean, so all the names, forms, and qualities of the universe are nothing other than Chiti. This world, which is full of Consciousness and is the body of Chiti at play, is no different from you, as the cool touch of water is no different from water. From an empirical point of view, cloth is simply cotton, and there cannot be any cloth without the cotton. From a spiritual point of view, the universe, though it may be seen with the eyes, is Brahman, and there cannot be any universe without Brahman. The universe is the play of its Creator; it is the play of the universal Consciousness. To see it like this is the worship of Parashakti, the true knowledge received from the Guru.

Those who are ignorant of this *chitshakti vilas,* this divine play of Consciousness, and consider the world to be different from Chiti, have to suffer in many ways because of this delusion. But those who see this Chiti-filled universe as Her game themselves become Chiti. This is also the teaching of Vedanta:

> *hai brahma sachchā jagat mithyā, yah mātra siddhānta hai*
> *brahmātmā ko jāne binū hotā nahim duḥkha kā anta hai*
> *jo jānatā saba mem eka ko vahī nara pātā śānti hai*
> *jo brahma hai so ātma hai yahī kahatā vedānta hai*

The Absolute is real, the world is unreal: this is the only truth. Without knowledge of the absolute Self there is no end to suffering. He who knows the One in all attains peace. The Absolute is the individual soul—this is what Vedanta says.

Siddha students should contemplate the preceding great mantra and thereby become aware of their own true nature.

A true leader of India, who has a strong feeling of identity and intimacy with India and her people, will automatically experience the nondual feeling that "I am the soul of India; India is my very soul" arising within him night and day, while getting up, sitting down, coming and going, whatever he may be doing. A member of a large, long-established family, with a hundred or two hundred members, big and small, will look upon them all as one, saying, "This family is mine," in spite of the fact that he has his own personal world of brothers, children, and grandchildren. In the same way, dear Siddha students, you should let your hearts beat spontaneously night and day with thoughts of supreme Shiva: "Shiva is mine, I am Shiva's. The universe He made is Shiva, all its movements are Shiva, and He is no different from me."

yah viśva śiva kī vāṭikā hai sair karne ke liye
nā rāga īrṣyā dveṣa chintā vair karne ke liye
yah viśva śiva kī mūrti śiva-bhakti karne ke liye
viśva śabda kā bādha kara śiva-dhyāna karne ke liye
yah viśva śiva-avatār hai na jāna dhokhā khāya hai
śiva se vilakshaṇa jāna kar vyartha atibhaya pāya hai
yah viśva śiva-darpaṇa bhavan śiva bana jo bhītara dekhatā
sarvatra hī śiva eka usako bimba pratibimba bhāsatā

This universe is Shiva's garden, meant for roaming in,
Not for attachment, jealousy, aversion, anxiety or enmity.
This universe is the image of Shiva, meant for his worship;
Destroy the concept "universe" and meditate on Shiva.
This universe is the incarnation of Shiva. If you do not know
       this, you are deceived.
If you consider it different from Shiva, you become terrified
       without reason.
This universe is a mansion containing the mirror of Shiva.
Whoever looks in it feeling one with Shiva, sees His own
       images and reflections,
Sees Shiva everywhere.

Now I give another mantra for Siddha students to think about:

> *sarvo mamāyaṁ vibhava ityevaṁ parijānataḥ*
> *viśvātmano vikalpānāṁ prasare'pi maheśatā*
>
>   (*Ishvarapratyabhijna*)

He who knows all this glory of manifestation as his own, who
realizes the entire cosmos in his Self, is divine, even though
thoughts may play in his mind.

Dear Siddha students, you should assimilate the essence and
achieve the fruit of the mantra by putting it into practice. A man
who can see his own identity with the universe, this assembly of thirty-
six elements, which is perceived through the senses and which supports
and sustains our life, saying, "This is my splendor and my glory," will
never lose his divinity and perfection. Even though he retains the
mind's tendency to see multiplicity and differentiation where non-
duality and identity really exist, this perfection will not be disturbed.

Just as the Pacific Ocean remains an ocean even when it breaks into waves, in the same way, as long as you are aware that the whole universe is your own splendor, you will realize your Godhood, and remain in that realization despite your tendency to see the universe as separate from yourself.

O Siddha students, the universe is yours. You are the soul of the universe. The changes, permutations, and combinations of the universe arise from you. They are yours. As the soul of the universe you are perfect. Keep on remembering that the universe is your own grandeur. This is the Guru's teaching to you, the teaching of Parashiva and the rule of the Siddhas. It is the easy and natural way to liberation. It is the holy sacrifice to please Parashakti. It is the great mantra for merging in Chiti. It is knowledge of the Self. It is meditation on the Guru. It is the sacrifice which fulfills Muktananda's own sacred duty.

Book Two
Teachings of the Siddhas

One

The Command of the Siddhas

Dear Siddha students, I have something important to tell you. Our way is the way of the Siddhas. Our tradition is the tradition of the Siddhas. Our world is the world of the Siddhas. Our beloved Gurus live in Siddhaloka. Our mantra is the Siddha mantra. Our system and rules are also those of the Siddhas. Our lives are under the protection of the Siddhas. Our *sadhana* is that of the Siddhas. Our goal is self-realization. We are to live as Siddhas, and we are to go to Siddhaloka. Everything that we do becomes perfect, for the grace of a Siddha is never without fruit; it is unfailing.

Fish fry have all the characteristics of fish, even though they are small, and they live very naturally in water. A lion cub is a lion in every way. An elephant calf is still an elephant, even though it may not have tusks. It has the same fluids, blood, intelligence, teeth, bones, and flesh as the one that gave birth to it, even though it is young. In exactly the same way, you carry within you the perfection of your perfect Father. So you do not have to think about it. There is nothing for you to worry about. A child grows naturally in the course of time, with the passing of the years. It is pointless for him to wonder, "Why is my ear small? Why don't I have any teeth? Why don't people think I'm big? Why don't I have the abilities that grown-ups have?" As you grow day by day, all the potential inherent in the seed of your father will be realized. A human being naturally grows from childhood to full youth, so it is foolish and confusing to worry about whether or not it is going to happen. This foolishness is an obstacle. You should not let such anxieties weaken your patience and strength. Remember that a Siddha's disciple can never remain in bondage.

Young Siddha students should follow their parents' advice. It is necessary for them to live under their control. It is necessary that Siddha students be regular and disciplined; otherwise they will not get the full benefit of their *sadhana*. Their *sadhana* will be weakened, they will fall short of perfection, and their growth will be obstructed. It will take longer for them to become one with Chiti.

A lion cub can never really be like a donkey; in its claws, its head —its whole body—it is completely a lion. But if it were to spend all its time with donkeys, it would start to lose its bravery, and the donkeys would begin to think it was one of them. It would gradually change its own spirit, its nature, and its habits, and take on the characteristics of a donkey. It would start to bray like a donkey, eat filthy things, and bathe in dirty water in the streets, as donkeys do. If it did this for long, then only its body would be a lion's; all its inner characteristics would be a donkey's. It would slowly forget its bravery and courage, its love of the forest solitude, its species, its habits, and all the ways of a lion. It would live in the streets of villages and towns. And then one day a washerman would come along looking for a beast to carry the dirty clothes of the town, and along with all the donkeys, the lion would have to journey to and from the washing place carrying dirty clothes. But it would never think it was a lion that had turned into a donkey. It would think that, since donkeys are in the majority, it had improved on its own species.

It is progress when a donkey turns into a lion, not when a lion turns into a donkey. Siddha students should not wander aimlessly from one place to another, from one house to another, like bound seekers, enduring slight and scorn. Your domain, Siddhaloka, is the greatest of all. It is a world of enormous power. Compared with this world of yours, Indraloka, Chandraloka, Suryaloka, and all the other worlds are worth nothing. You belong to a noble family, and countless Siddha yogis and yoginis of this family are standing behind you, protecting you. So don't waste your time with *sadhus* and devotees who are still ignorant. Remember that you have to go to Siddhaloka.

There are many, many of your predecessors living in Siddhaloka.

All Siddhas—from the supremely perfect primordial Lord Shiva and the Seven Sages, to the innumerable Siddha seers who have appeared since the earliest time—live in Siddhaloka possessing all their powers. They grant you Shakti, activate your yoga *sadhana*, and are always ready to protect you, to obtain what you need and preserve what you already have. You should not feel that you are the student of your Guru alone. You are a true descendant of the line of the inhabitants of Siddhaloka. You do not know your ancestry, but when you visit Siddhaloka, you will gain a full knowledge of your lineage. In your family there is, first of all, the primordial Shiva, the wise, the blissful, the great Lord. Then there are Narada, the sage of the gods, and the great sage Vyasa. There are also Shesha, Shukadeva, Yajnavalkya, Kakabhushandi, Suta, Shaunaka, Shandilya, Bhishma, and King Janaka. There are the milkmaids of Vraja, who all attained perfection, and such kings as Prithu, Ambarisha, and Bharata. Then there are countless other perfect beings, such as Prahlada, Dhruva, Sanaka, Hanuman, Akrura, Uddhava, Vidura, Sanjaya, Sudama, Kasyapa, Satapa, Prishni, Manu, Dasharatha, Kaushalya, and King Vibhishana. Belonging to our times are Sai Baba of Shirdi, my beloved Zipruanna of Nasirabad, and your Paramaguru, Bhagavan Sri Nityananda. In Siddhaloka there are millions and millions of Siddha yogis and yoginis to protect you. So do not falter or hesitate in any way, but stay firm and steadfast in the Siddha Marga, with absolute faith and devotion.

It is because you do not know your own perfection that you look here and there. You must have a real and unswerving faith in your tradition, in the Siddha Path, in the yoga of meditation, and in the Siddha mantras. The grace of the Siddhas is behind you like a mountain, so why should you run here and there and destroy your firm faith? A faithful wife thinks of nothing but her husband. She loves only him; her religion is devotion to him; her needs are fulfilled when his needs are fulfilled; she rejoices in him alone, he is her only delight; her mantra is her husband; she surrenders her intellect to him; her wisdom, meditation, and her place of pilgrimage are him; the vow of her life is love of him; her addiction is to him; she is helpless without him. Siddha students, too, should be completely possessed with delight and love for the way of the Siddhas.

Do not worry that you have not achieved anything. It takes only a second for a Siddha to open you. When you have complete devotion and faith, a firm and devout will, and the readiness to surrender everything, then the grace of a Siddha will not be long in coming. You will receive it at once. When you receive the grace of a great Siddha, you become not only a liberated being who has completed his *sadhana*, but a full Siddha. A *sadhaka* becomes a Siddha through the grace of a Siddha. He can never remain in bondage. You should always be thinking of your Siddhaloka, of the divine capacity of Siddhas to turn the incompetent into the competent, of the light shining within you, and of the mantra of Consciousness that will raise you to Siddhahood. You should always remember that the great Shakti, who freely performs countless types of functions, is active within you, that the divine, radiant, and great Shakti is incarnate within you. You should realize your true worth and set your daily routine accordingly. Do not worry about what will happen to your *sadhana*, about when it will bear fruit or how complete are your attainments. As I have just said, a lion cub is always a lion. Pay special attention to this. This is the word of the Guru. This is obedience to the command of the Guru.

After listening to the entire *Gita*, Arjuna simply said: *karisye vachanam tava*—"I shall do Thy bidding." In the same way, you should obey the Guru's command completely. You should keep his teachings in your heart and follow the path he has shown you. This is the boat that will carry you across the ocean of worldly existence. With the same speed that you faithfully and lovingly take to heart the Guru's discipline, his commands, his teachings, and the path he shows you, you will receive the complete reward. Never disparage the Guru. This will deflect you from your *sadhana* and lead you into delusion. If there is enmity, jealousy, falsehood, and gossip among brother disciples so that the code of conduct of the Guru's family is broken, and if instead of meditating and studying you allow your minds to become agitated by quarrels, then the inner Shakti will gradually become weakened. Weeping, shouting, conceit, and hurting other people are not the marks of service to the Guru. Whenever my Gurudev called me, no matter how far away I was, I would rush to him saying, "Yes, Gurudev," three times. If he ever asked me anything, I would reply immediately because I did not want to trouble or annoy him by making him ask me again and again.

There is one thing that you must remember: the Shakti that is active and growing within you is the Guru himself. You should therefore be careful about the company you keep so that the purity of your *sadhana* is maintained. Bad company is dangerous, even fatal, so make a firm resolve to avoid it. When a man keeps the wrong company, all the bad features of a demon are automatically fostered in him, and he behaves like a demon. The noble qualities are destroyed. Kaikeyi, who was full of love, affection, and modesty, became the cause of grief to King Dasharatha, Bharata, and all the citizens of Ayodhya because of the evil influence of her maid Manthara, and she was forced to abandon her own beloved son Bharata. Just as a drop of sour curd can spoil a whole ocean of milk, so bad company can lead to every kind of evil. It can make you gossip about everyone and talk ill of them; it can make you indiscreet, arrogant, impure, full of animosity; it can make you behave dishonestly; it can draw you to movies and plays and to eat impure food in restaurants. Siddha students must be extremely careful to avoid bad company, for it reduces the momentum of the inner Shakti.

When Chiti Shakti opens Her eyes, the universe is born, and when She closes them, it is destroyed. When this same divine Chiti lives within you as your best friend, when She is working within you, when even the briefest meeting with Her makes everything full of warmth and happiness, you must understand how detrimental it would be to forsake Her friendship and Her delight and indulge in low company.

This instruction has been written under the inspiration of Chiti, is dear to Chiti, has been revealed from within Chiti, has arisen from the attainment of Chiti, is a theme pleasing to Chiti Shakti, is not different from Chiti, and is permeated by Chiti. To obey it is to attain Chiti.

Two

The Siddha Student's Awareness in the World

Dear Siddha students, I have been telling you over and over again that the world is nothing but the play of Chiti. When Chiti playfully expresses Herself in the form of universal Consciousness, She becomes the world, vibrating and creating innumerable world forms.

> *chideva bhagavatī svachchhasvatantrarūpā*
> *tattadanantajagadātmanā sphuratī*
>
> *(Pratyabhijnahridayam)*

It is the divine Consciousness alone, luminous, absolute, and free willed, which flashes forth in the form of numerous worlds.

When, through the yoga of meditation, the Siddha student attains this knowledge of Chiti, he sees the entire world, inner and outer, as Her play, sees Her vibrating in every action, and finds supreme joy in all his work and activities. This is because, through his insight, the Siddha student is constantly and completely aware of the expansion of Chiti. He knows that everything that happens in the world, because it is the flowering of Chiti, is Chiti. With this knowledge that everything is the divine Chiti, he understands that the inner satisfaction that comes even from such mundane things as eating, drinking, and enjoying oneself is a blissful impulse of Chiti, and so he himself becomes full of bliss. With a mind made pure through meditating on Chiti, he realizes that the enjoyment arising from the sense pleasures appropriate to his particular stage in life is no different from Chiti. Not only this; just as he feels satisfied and happy in his enjoyment of the pleasures of the senses, so he enjoys the same bliss of Chiti when he is without them. Such a yogi of the world sees everything in the world as the doing of Chiti, understands that the movement which throbs in everything is the vibration of the blissful Chiti, and thus his mind becomes completely satisfied. As this state of satisfaction is continually being consolidated through the strength of his contemplation, his mind gradually sheds it doubts and imaginings, and the light of supreme bliss spreads within him. The *Vijnanabhairava* says:

> *jagdhipānakrutollāsarasānandavi jrumbhaṇāta*
> *bhāvayedbharitāvasthāṁ mahānandamayo bhavet*
> *gītādiviṣayāsvādāsamasaukhyaikatātmanaḥ*
> *yoginastanmayatvena manorūḍhestadātmatā*
> *yatra yatra manastuṣṭirmanastatraiva dhārayet*
> *tatra tatra parānandasvarūpaṁ samprakāśate*

When one experiences the joy that spreads from the savor arising from the pleasure of eating and drinking, one should contemplate the perfect condition of that joy; then one would become saturated with great bliss. When a yogi identifies himself with the incomparable joy of song or other things, this concentrated yogi becomes one with that joy. Wherever the mind finds its satisfaction, let it be concentrated on that. In every case the true nature of the highest bliss will shine forth.

The truth is that suffering is not knowing the Lord God who pervades the world, while happiness is knowing Him. Dear Siddha students, you are conscious, all-pervasive, and perfect. The universe is not at all different from you. What is it that you want to renounce? What are you running after to possess? There is nothing in the world but you. It is you who pervade the universe, who are the perfect and undying principle. There is no difference between you and the world. There is no duality. You fill the whole universe, without differentiation. You are the serene, imperishable, and pure Kundalini, the light of Consciousness. There never was and never will be any ignorance in you. You are the play of universal Consciousness. You are not *rajasic* or *tamasic*; you are not dominated by any particular element. You are *nirguna* and *saguna*. God without form and God with form. You are the untainted and unchangeable play of pure Chiti. Golden bangles, bracelets, anklets, and necklaces are all gold; in the same way, the world born from the blossoming forth of the Shakti of Parashiva is nothing other than Chiti. The effect cannot run counter to the cause.

Dear Siddha students! Wherever you look, whatever you see, is all your own light. Nothing is different from you. You are present in everything. You should not think of such distinctions as, "I am here, I am not there." Instead, your constant meditation should be the thought, "I am everywhere, I am the Self of all." Nothing other than you exists in the world. The *Shiva Sutras* say: *svaśaktiprachayo'sya viśvam*—"The universe is the expansion of one's own Shakti." The illusion called the universe has arisen in you solely through your own mental impurities. Worship Goddess Chiti, and as you become free from impurities, the universe will appear as the resting place of Chiti. You are pure Consciousness; you are pure Reality. The whole visible universe is a vibration of you. Why are you afflicted when there is no reason for it? Everything is saturated with Chiti. You were real in the very beginning, you are real now, and you will remain real forever. You do not actually come and go. You are not in bondage, so where is the question of being liberated? Chiti does everything, so how can you be the experiencer? You are everywhere in your fullness; you are the ever-blissful Reality. Do not let your mind get caught up in the conflicts of desires and doubts. Understand that these too are the vibrations of Chiti, and let them dissolve in Her. You should understand that there is perfection even in what may appear to be imperfect. Let your desires become filled with Chiti, and so live your life without desire. Let the object of meditation in the heart become all-pervading, let it spread everywhere. The Self is forever perfect—realize that, and make the meditator the object of meditation. Since there is no "other," what is there to meditate on? See your own glory everywhere, and so fill your mind with peace. You may have spent your whole life reflecting on the meaning of the scriptures, or teaching people about the six schools of philosophy, or preaching sermons, but as long as you have not become one with Chiti, your fear will never leave you.

When the differentiating mentality that sees "I and mine" is burned away in the fire of meditation, you will find supreme and undying bliss.

You can perform any number of noble deeds, enjoy any number of pleasures, go into *samadhi* a million times, but as long as you are different from Chiti you will never achieve release from bondage. When you merge with Chiti you will find undying joy. "I have to do this, I shouldn't do this, I have done this much, this much is left to be done" —free yourself from all these dualities. Give up religious bigotry. Renounce your desires, even the desire for liberation. Give up all expectations and enter into the repose of Chiti. In Her you will find unconditional peace and undying happiness. A man who renounces sense objects cannot forget his antagonism toward them; a man who embraces them becomes bound by his love of them. Beloved Siddha students! Do not become attached to sense objects, and do not become disgusted by them. Only then can you become *muktananda*, one who possesses the joy of freedom, unentangled in conflicts and dualities, enjoying everlasting peace.

As long as "possession and renunciation" control you, you will still be bound to the world. While they exist the world will exist for you, but a man who forgets about "possession and renunciation" goes beyond worldly existence. Neither renounce "possession-renunciation" nor accept it. Become absorbed in your inner reality. Think of the world as the play of Chitshakti and find true peace. If you can always be aware of Chiti when you are hearing, seeing, touching, smelling, eating, drinking, waking, and sleeping, you will never be depressed or sad. Such a Siddha student is perpetually liberated. The wise man who is unattached like the sky and never at any time allows his mind to become agitated has perfected his meditation, for he has become one with Chiti. He is extremely fortunate. The man who is asleep to the world but awake to contemplation of the Self will enjoy supreme bliss forever. The Siddha student who is filled with eternal bliss, with *Nityananda,* is fully worthy. He is great. The Siddha student who knows his true nature and remains absorbed in his Self, who lives in close contact with his inner being and finds contentment there, who feels neither distaste for crowds nor any special taste for solitude, is a great and holy center of the pilgrimage.

The whole world is simply an illusion. From the point of view of ultimate reality, it is the play of Chiti. The eternal and everlasting reality of Shiva pulsates throughout the entire universe. The Siddha student who knows that everything is the pure light of Consciousness, composed of the red, white, black, and Blue lights, is himself the very image of Chiti. He has completed his *sadhana*. He has achieved nonattachment to differentiation, renunciation, and forms. He has heard, reflected on, and contemplated Mother Chiti and established Her in his heart. The enlightened man who knows directly the identity of the Self and the Absolute is a true Siddha student. He is blessed and worthy of being honored by the world. He has recognized his own Self in the many different forms. He is no longer concerned with the body or anything else. He considers everything as *chitshakti vilas*, the play of the divine Consciousness. He is established in wisdom, ever free; he has found the divine joy of the Absolute. Such a Siddha student is liberated while still in the body.

The mother and father of such a one are also blessed. He lives with his family without being attached to them. He regards alike both praise and censure. He accepts worldly pleasures when they come to him, but he is not attracted to sensuality. A person whose mind is free of desires and whose vision is filled with Chiti is liberated while still in the body.

He does not see the universe as the universe, for he knows that it is solely the play of Chiti Shakti. He sees the light of Chiti in friend, in enemy, in all beings. He worships the whole universe as God. Such a one is liberated, even while living in the world. He lives with everybody and yet is associated with nobody. He is dyed so deeply in the color of Chiti that no other color can affect him. He is drunk with his own Self. He is in love with his own Self. He is content with his own Self. He is forever liberated while still in the body.

He leads his day-to-day life in the world normally, and even though he may appear agitated, inside he is supremely peaceful. In his attachment there is no attachment; in his aversion there is no aversion. He is free from all *gunas*; he loves all beings. He is easily liberated while still in the body.

He is never upset by suffering, nor does he desire happiness. He never leaves the path of virtue; he never follows the path of evil. His mind is always filled with the vibrations of Chiti. He is profound, steadfast, pure, and detached. He is compassionate, loving, and gracious. Such a Siddha student is liberated while living in the world.

He is not afraid of death, nor does he take much interest in life. For him, life and death are both the play of Chiti. He knows the Chiti Shakti completely. He attains the full grace of Sri Gurudev. Such an enlightened one is said to be liberated while still in the world.

For him there is no *maya* and no body; the universe is the garden of Chiti. He knows that God is the individual soul as well as the world. Such an enlightened Siddha student finds full repose in the Goddess Chiti. Born as a human being, he has done what he had to do. There is nothing else for him to accomplish, nothing else for him to attain. He has found all that he had to find. He has understood that which had to be understood: his own Self. He has found Shiva within his own Self. He is Vaikuntha, Kailasa, Badrinath, Kashi. All holy places are where he is.

Three
Pretense of Meditation

Dear Siddha students! Your meditation should be genuine. Hypocrites and cheats meditate just for praise or to feed their own reputations. If you do this, you are just deceiving yourself—picking your own pocket—and what's the use of that? When a hypocrite is put to the test, it is hard for him to get through it.

It's very good if you're having a lot of *kriyas;* your meditation should be full of intense feeling. But take care that you don't allow any ulterior motive to get into this feeling. Yogis of meditation! You should store up the wealth of the inner Shakti instead of external riches. The inner Shakti is all-knowing and wise. The Shakti knows when you are full of feeling, and that finds expression through *kriyas.* She possesses full knowledge of the *kriyas* and events of the past, present, and future, for She is no different from the omniscient Shiva. According to the *Spandakarika: seyaṁ kriyātmikā śaktiḥ śivasya paśuvartinī*—"It is the Shakti of Shiva that underlies the *kriyas* and is embodied in living creatures." The same Shakti of Parashiva is active in you. This same Shakti lives in the supreme Guru Nityananda. O Siddha students! You should be sure that your *sadhana* path is good, that it is authentic, because as your inner Self, the Shaki underlying these *kriyas* sees everything.

I know a good yogi who gives Shaktipat. He has everybody meditate standing up in a line, and when they are all lined up and ready, he says the words, "I give." At this, everybody is strongly affected, and they begin doing all sorts of *kriyas.* Some people weep, some laugh, some cry out, and some dance. After an hour of this, he says, "I take," and they all come out of meditation and return to their normal state. If someone does not come out of meditation, the yogi has to say to him, "Come out, Madhavji; come out, Uddhavji," and the person is not considered ready for meditation. That yogi says, "*Kriyas* take place when I give the Shakti of my own accord by saying, 'I give.' When I take the Shakti back by saying, 'I take,' and someone doesn't come out of meditation, then that person is meditating not because of the force of the Shakti but because he is a fraud and a hypocrite."

There are many people who tell each other, "I had such a wonderful meditation. I had such wonderful feelings. It was so marvelous." They say this simply because they want praise. Their meditation is for applause and is not the meditation of the Self. The poets call this meditation "heron meditation."

The heron shuts his eyes and stands in a lake, pond, or running stream, meditating for hours on end. He spends his whole life like this, standing in meditation for long periods every day. Yet he has not received Shaktipat or seen the inner lights or realized God. This is because he does not meditate on God, but on fish. He does not meditate for the peace of the Self, but in order to kill fish to fill his stomach. He practices the meditation of nourishing the body by eating good fish. It is a meditation of enjoyment and pleasure. If someone said to me, "Babaji, there are lots of herons meditating in the river over there, and they never leave the place, so why don't they get the rewards of meditation, namely, bliss, the vision of lights, and *samadhi*?" I would say to them, "What a good question you have asked. How clever you are, how wise, how perceptive. Who knows what a high state you have reached! However, you are talking like a blind man and a fool. Look brother, the heron meditates to catch fish, to eat and enjoy them, and to make himself strong." There are yogis just like the heron; they do not meditate on Sadguru Nityananda or the divine Shakti. These heron students do not meditate on the nature of their own Self but on fish, and that's what they get. One who meditates on fish will always catch fish and eat fish and be peaceful and contented. Tell me, can you find God if you meditate on fish? Can you see the inner lights if you meditate on fish? You meditate on snack bars and films, and yet you want *samadhi*! Meditating yogis, you won't find paradise through heron meditation because you find whatever you meditate on.

If Siddha students were to understand the Guru's Shakti, they would be saved from this artificial heron meditation. The Shakti that brings them meditation works in them in five forms, which are described in the *Tantrasara* as follows:

> *prakāśarūpatā chitśaktiḥ svātantryam ānandaśaktiḥ*
> *tatchamatkāra ichchhāśaktiḥ āmarṣātmakatā jnānaśaktiḥ*
> *sarvākārayogitvaṁ kriyāśaktiḥ*

The power of intelligence, or pure light of intelligence is *chitshakti*; the power of will is *ichchashakti*; the power of realizing absolute bliss is *anandashakti*; the power of knowledge is *jnanashakti*; the power of creating is *kriyashakti*.

This means that the Chitshakti enters you from Sri Gurudev with Her supreme radiance and Her independent joy; She performs countless miracles out of Her own free will; She knows everything in your heart, great and small; She knows which yogic *kriyas* are necessary and should occur in your particular case, and She causes these *kriyas* to happen. In other words, the supreme Shakti of the one Parashiva, whom we call Chiti Shakti Kundalini, the Shakti of the Guru's grace or the Guru's own spiritual power, lives within you in Her five aspects: consciousness, bliss, volition, knowledge, and action. Chiti Shakti lives in the same form in the immanent Shiva and in the transcendent supreme Shiva, and She lives in the same measure within your Guru. Furthermore, that which is in your Guru is naturally in you. So if you belong to the Guru and stay his, the Shakti will be in you to the same degree. This Shakti is not present in heron meditation.

The Shakti does not depend on any support. She is self-effulgent. She freely enjoys Her own bliss within Herself and needs nothing else. She is the power of will, resolute and unique, who can perform any miracle She desires. She is the power of knowledge acting within both the knower and the known. She is the power of action who produces the energy which creates the innumerable objects of the world. This fivefold Shakti is in God; the same Shakti is in every Guru. It enters each disciple according to his worth. The same fivefold Shakti pervades as one force the disciple, the Guru, and God. Unless you realize this, you will not understand how the Guru knows the quality of your meditation and the feelings of your heart. This is why I say that you should never let yourself get into heron meditation.

The heron stands in a lake from morning to evening with his eyes shut, but he does not find the light of Chiti Shakti. He does not experience the happiness of the power of bliss, nor the miracles of the power of volition, nor the fruit of the discriminating power of knowledge, nor the direct experience of the power of action. Why not? Because, although it looks like a yogi's meditation, the heron's meditation is on fish. What results do you want from meditation? What do you contemplate in meditation? You meditate for a set period, but what does your mind actually love? You see someone crying, so you cry, but you don't know why he is crying. You see someone laughing, so you laugh, but you don't know why he is laughing. Someone is waving a finger, so you wave ten, but you don't know why he is doing it or why you are doing it. Someone spins around once, so you spin around twenty-five times. But you don't know why he is spinning or why you spin around so many times. You are only imitating him. His movements are caused by the inner Shakti, but yours are caused by your external mind. This is what is called heron meditation. Muktananda says to both, "Well done. What fine *kriyas* you are having. You've come a long way. You've risen very high. How wonderful." He blesses both of them like this. A heron meditates all day on fish and fills his stomach with fish. You have laughed a little, cried a little, done some *kriyas,* and have been congratulated tenfold for all this. So what else should happen? The heron meditates on fish, and you meditate on praise, not on the inner Shakti. The heron gets fish; you get praise. If anyone asks you and the heron why you haven't reached Vaikuntha, the answer will be that you never meditated on Vaikuntha. You receive what you meditate on.

There are many ashrams that grant you the fruit of your desires. About twenty years ago I lived near an ashram that contained the *samadhi* shrine of a Siddha saint. Many pilgrims would visit this *samadhi.* I also used to go. I would walk around the tomb solely out of devotion for the Self. Then I would meditate quietly in a distant corner; my mind would contemplate the Self, and so I obtained the fruit of this practice. Among the other people who habitually visited the *samadhi* was a married couple. They had no children, and they used to sit down and meditate because they wanted a child. Eventually they received some instructions, and a child was born to them. There was also a man who came because he wanted to win a court case, another who came because he wanted to pass his college exams, and another who came because he wanted to get rid of an illness. There were people who came to meditate because they wanted to make money and people who came to meditate in order to satisfy their sensuous desires. There were also those people who came simply for leisure and enjoyment and who used the *samadhi* as a rendezvous, since it was not easy for them to meet in Bombay. They would make an agreement, "You come from that direction, I'll come from this direction." In particular, college boys and girls would make pilgrimages to the *samadhi* to meet in secret, for no one is forbidden to visit a *samadhi.* Thus, many people, including Swami Muktananda, used to visit this place.

People would say, "Muktananda Swami received *siddhis* at the *samadhi.* Why didn't other people get anything from the shrine of the Baba?" Then they would say to me, "Swamiji, why did you get so much when other people didn't get anything?"

I would reply, "They got everything too. I got what I wanted. I wanted knowledge, meditation, devotion, and close friendship with God, and these things were granted to me. The couple who wanted a child, got a child; the man who wanted knowledge got knowledge; the man who wanted to win his court case won his court case; the man who wanted health became healthy, and the boys and girls who wanted to carry on their love affairs carried on their love affairs. Everyone got just what they wanted."

You will get the fruit of your meditation in different ways and in varying degrees according to the depth of your feelings, your basic nature, your faith in the Guru and your knowledge of him, your faith in the inner Shakti and your knowledge of Her ways, the manner in which you meditate, and the motives behind your meditation. If, like a heron, you are only pretending to meditate, a flying chariot will not descend from Mount Kailasa. However, you will certainly get a couple of fish to eat. Therefore, in meditation you should be careful, and your desire should be pure.

You must see where it is that your mind concentrates itself, how involved it gets in other things. When Muktananda meditated, he had one supreme deity: Bhagavan Nityananda. Nityananda was his Guru-brother and his Guru-sister. He did not give his love to any Guru-brother or have a relationship with any Guru-sister. After all, what's the use of finding new brothers and sisters when you have left your real ones? Isn't there deceit and falsehood in such relationships? All the people in the world are one's brothers and sisters, and there's no value in becoming attached to one and averse to another. Nityananda was Muktananda's dear relative and friend. He had no friends besides him, and he never deceived anyone in the name of Nityananda. He constantly meditated on Nityananda, reflected on Nityananda, thought about Nityananda. In Nityananda he found complete satisfaction. In him he found full contentment, peace, joy, and Self-knowledge.

One day when I went into the meditation room in the Ashram, I found a young yogini laughing loudly, her eyes closed in a charming *mudra.* I went over to her and said, "You seem very happy. Why are you laughing so much?"

She answered, "Baba, I was just thinking that some people believe you're simple-minded. They think they can fool you and trick you by pretending to meditate with great intensity. However, you are neither fooled nor tricked. You pretend that you don't know what's going on and bluff them. That's what's making me laugh."

I said, "Daughter, its very true. I give them just what they want."

Meditators! You may be meditating very deeply, having *kriyas* and experiencing all sorts of deep and intense feelings, but remember that within me the power of knowledge which is also your own inner Self is ready with paper and pencil to give a "report" on all of this. This girl was quite right to laugh and say what she did. It was her remark that inspired me to write this chapter. It was this power that revealed the above secret to her. I have a sort of secret "meditation meter" that nobody can see, but with it I can see what kind of meditation you are doing and what your real worth is. Therefore, examine yourselves and see what type of outer and inner *kriyas* you have. Toward what goal are your actions directed? How much inner faith do you have? What does your mind cling to or seek refuge in? This will indicate your real motives for visiting the sacred shrine—whether you're seeking children, a cure for a disease, employment, or a college degree. Whatever desire there may be behind your pilgrimage, that will be fulfilled. So examine thoroughly your motives for meditating. You ask me why you don't see Rameshwaram when your thoughts are directed north. O brother! Rameshwaram is in the south. Turn yourself around. Meditate on the south. Then you will see Rameshwaram. I have a great desire to tell a story for today's pilgrims on the spiritual path. It is the story of Laila and Majnu, taken from the discourses of Swami Ram Tirtha.

Laila was the daughter of a king, and Majnu was the son of a laborer. They were very much in love but could not get married because of the difference in their social status. This, however, did not prevent them yearning for each other with deep love. Their love increased every day until they became almost mad thinking about each other. Laila would climb to a room high up in the palace and call, "Majnu, Majnu." Majnu would wander through the streets of the city, crying "Laila, Laila." He had only one ambition—to be united with Laila. She was his only desire, his only succor, his only hope. Majnu was not promiscuous for a moment; he did not think of anything but Laila. When Majnu's father saw his son's madness, he was very frightened, thinking that the king would punish Majnu. But Majnu himself was not frightened, for true love does not care about anything.

The king, Laila's father, was also very worried when he saw his daughter's condition. He called doctors, magicians, astrologers, and experts in mantras and *tantras,* but nothing had any effect on her. He would suggest a visit to the theater to divert her, but she would only say, "Will Majnu be there?"

He would say, "Let us travel far away into a cool and beautiful land."

She would reply, "Majnu is not there. I don't want to go." Thus Majnu and Laila pined for each other. Muktananda says: If you long for something, long for it like this, otherwise don't. To pursue something for selfish ends is of no use and cannot lead you to God.

Because they thought about each other and meditated on each other all the time, Laila and Majnu completely lost themselves. Laila thought about Majnu so much that she became Majnu, and Majnu thought about Laila so much that he became Laila. If a meditator withholds a part of himself and does not lose himself completely, he is a thief; he is stealing what he holds back. A poem I once heard describes Majnu's state exactly:

> *khaṭakā nahīṁ hai khāne kā chintā nahīṁ hai pāne kī*
> *mamatā nahīṁ hai deha kī paravāha nahīṁ hai prāṇoṅ kī*

He is not worried about his food nor anxious for any gain;
He is not attached to his body, nor does he cling to life itself.

Majnu had only one hope—that he might attain Laila. He wandered around completely forgetful of himself. The people of the city took him for a lunatic. Seeing Majnu in this state, the king felt pity for him, for he became convinced that Majnu's love for his daughter was true. Majnu had ceased to exist as Majnu and had offered himself to Laila, like earrings melting into gold. He saw Laila everywhere he looked. There was no more "you and I"; only Laila remained. The king ordered a proclamation in the town: "Majnu is not well. His love for Laila has made him helpless. Give him food and drink and clothes, and send the bills to the royal treasury." Everywhere in the town it was heard that Majnu, because he had thought about nothing but Laila, was to receive everything he wanted from the king. All the destitute, lazy, and needy people in the town—all the parasites—realized that it would be a good plan to pretend to be Majnu, and so every day a new Majnu appeared. The number of new Majnus increased.

All the new Majnus got shoes, clothes, and food from the shopkeepers, and the bills were sent to the treasury. The king noticed that Majnu's bills were running into thousands, and he had inquiries made. He discovered that there were over a thousand Majnus in the town. "Because I had pity this misfortune has come," he thought to himself, wondering what to do next. He had a very clever minister in his service and this minister said, "Your Majesty, if you delegate full authority to me, I shall handle the matter." The king agreed, and the minister sent the crier around to proclaim: "Exactly one week from today, at 12:00 noon, Majnu will be hanged, for he has fallen in love with the princess and this is against the law." The effect of this proclamation was startling. All the Majnus threw away their clothes and shoes and hats and ran as far away as they could. They found jobs in offices and houses and factories. They all did their best to hide their identities since if they were discovered they would be hanged. All of them disappeared. Only the real Majnu remained. He was quite ready to be speared to death or burned alive, for he had no desire to keep his life. His only desire was for Laila. He had lost himself in Laila. Only the real Majnu had a genuine desire, and only he was left. And it was the real Majnu who found his Laila.

Dear students of meditation! Your worth can only be ascertained when your are put through a test, and there is a test for meditation, just as there is for anything else. The one who proves to be a true Majnu, a true meditator, will find his Laila, which is God. The rest will throw off their clothes and shoes and hats and run away. The state of a true meditator is like the state of Majnu. Do real meditation instead of meditating like a heron. You will find true happiness.

Welcoming the fivefold Shakti within you, you should always think of the Guru and lose yourself in him. The man who loses his sense of himself through meditation and lets himself merge with his deity becomes that deity, just as an earring, when it is melted down, becomes a piece of gold. The man who merges into his deity attains Godhood. He is completely blessed, and his parents too are blessed. Only a man like this attains everlasting life: from a mortal he becomes immortal.

When a devotee receives the nectar of devotion, when he sees the world as empty and his own Self pervading all beings, from Brahman to an insect, then he becomes full of love within and without. Every hair of his body is filled with love. The Guru's knowledge will certainly be in one who has this sort of devotion. Chiti will play in him all the time. He is a worthy Siddha student, for he has really understood the greatness of meditation. He constantly honors the Guru Shakti revealed within him, and sings the praises of the Guru. All his weeping ceases. Muktananda says that a man like this has found complete and eternal bliss. Nityananda is truly within him.

Truth is rewarded with truth and falsehood with falsehood, and you must decide which you want. If you want Truth, meditate with truth. Perfect peace is not far away; it lies within your own Self. But first you must become completely pure.

Four

The Secret of Renunciation

It is certainly true that through renunciation one can find great peace. The Lord Himself says in the *Gita* (12:12): *tyāgāchchhāntiranantaram* —"Endless peace comes from renunciation." However, there are differences of opinion on the meaning of renunciation and on the order in which things should be renounced. Some people renounce their homes, but they still weep because they are without peace. Some renounce their religion, but they still weep due to lack of peace. Some give up their clothes, rub their bodies with sacred ash, and become known as ascetics, but still they do not find peace. Some give up food and drink milk. They are called "food renouncers." Some people renounce women, others their homes, others speech. But they are all still hungry for peace and have not attained any.

From this you can see that there are many types of renunciation. Every day renunciants find something new to renounce, but it is depression rather than peace that they attain. The Lord says that peace comes through renunciation, and that is true; the question is of what we should renounce and how we should renounce. Nowadays there is more ostentation than sincerity in renunciation. This irritates and frightens ordinary people. For them, piercing the ears and plucking out the hair are not devotion but just another nuisance.

Many people think that if you live an ordinary life in the world, there are no means for you to find peace. Renunciation is necessary, absolutely necessary. They think that if you want peace you must live in a cave or forest or on the top of a mountain and torture your body. These mistaken ideas about renunciation have spread all over the world; but the truth is that, through the yoga of meditation, it is possible for all people to quiet their minds.

There is another common misunderstanding among people who live in the world. They think they have a moral obligation to live only for their families, their houses, and a series of dreary pleasures, and that meditation, renunciation, and yoga are exclusively for *sadhus* and ascetics who have renounced their homes. But Muktananda says: Yoga, meditation, and renunciation are meant precisely for those who live in the world, who have wives, husbands, and families, who have factories and industries, wealth and property and homes. There is no doubt that renunciation is necessary, but what do we mean by renunciation? There are mendicants who wander around crying, "Renunciation, renunciation." There are innumerable sects who literally live on the label "renunciation," who use the word "renunciation" as a mantra, and who maintain their identities by means of the outer trappings of renunciation. But there is still no attainment of peace. Renunciation is essential if you want peace, but it has to be of the right kind. Krishnanath renounces Ramanath's hat, and then looks for the chariot from heaven as a reward for his renunciation. That is not renunciation.

A beloved devotee once gave me a book by an unknown Russian saint. It was excellent, but in describing how he sets off on his pilgrimage, the Russian yogi says, "I have become a complete renunciant. In my bag I have two pieces of bread and a Bible. I have a shawl to cover myself and that is all." In India too there are renunciants like this. These "complete renunciants" will only eat when the food is put right in their hands, and if it isn't, they stay hungry. Some even keep a man running after them from morning until night holding their food which, if they feel like it, they may decide to eat in the evening. Someone I knew met one of these renunciants, and he said to me, "He's such a great renunciant; he eats only if he is fed. He has half a dozen people around him to make sure he gets everything he needs." I replied, "Brother, I think I am more of a renunciant than he, and a more practical renunciant too. I have renounced the six men who are kept standing around to attend to the needs of one. I eat punctually every day and put the food in my mouth with my own hands. At the normal rate, each man must be paid two *rupees* a day. That means twelve *rupees* for all of them. Isn't it ludicrous to keep six men from their work and call yourself a renunciant? I eat without any help. Surely not to be dependent on half-a-dozen other people is renunciation." At this the man was silent.

There are many kinds of renunciation. But we should look at the people who practice renunciation and ask ourselves what they have gained from it. Where has that peace which the Lord says comes from renunciation disappeared? Senseless people's renunciation reaches its peak when they will only eat and drink when food and drink is given to them. What have they got out of all this? Where is that peace, that freedom of pure joy? A sensible man will use his brains about renunciation and ask himself what there is in this world that is really his own and which he is therefore at liberty to give up.

In India there is a form of worship in which an innocent sheep is brought before the Goddess and killed. The foolish people who practice this type of animal sacrifice offer the Goddess the head of the sheep and expect reward for themselves. This is a contemptible form of worship. It is a great pity that even the priest thinks that benefit can be gained by someone else's sacrifice. This kind of worship is completely senseless. One's renunciation has to be intelligent, honest, and properly thought out; otherwise it is of no value. If you leave your home to go and live in a monastery or in the jungle, then all you've done is change your house. If you give up white clothes and wear red ones, then all you've done is change the color of your clothes.

There was once an emperor of renunciants, King Shikhidhvaja. The story of his renunciation, which appears in the *Yoga Vasishtha*, is worth thinking about. The story of his renunciation is the story of a true awakening; it calms the mind and gives supreme peace. Although a king, Shikhidhvaja was a very religious man and an earnest seeker. He really wanted to realize the supreme truth. Day by day his longing increased. He used to see many saints, *mahatmas*, sages, and seers, and in addition to these faithful and devoted associations, he practiced *sadhana*. His aspiration grew all the time, and his yearning for God eventually became so strong that he felt desperate. Having tried various types of *sadhana*, he finally came to the conclusion that he would not attain anything without renunciation, that there could be no peace or equanimity without renunciation, and that renunciation was the most direct way to Truth for all times. He thought long and deeply about what should be renounced, and when and how he should renounce. He finally decided that he should first of all give up his throne.

He decided to entrust the throne to his queen and himself go to the forest. He called his beloved queen, Chudala, and told her everything that was in his heart. He said, "I can't live without the peace of the Self. My ignorant heart is always frightened by the world. It is only my pride in being a king that gives my life substance. When I sleep, I sleep like every man; and when I eat, I eat like every man. Is there anyone in the world who has not been devoured by time? How foolish it is that I still desire to live. Why shouldn't I give up this perishable and transient life now when I have to leave it after death anyway? O my Queen Chudala, my most beloved wife! You have done many things for me, and now I ask you to do one more. Take care of the kingdom so that I may go and find peace and contentment and put out the anguish in my soul."

The queen knew perfectly well what was going on in King Shikhidhvaja's mind. She had followed the path taught her by her Guru and had perfected the yoga of meditation, through which she had gained the knowledge of past, present, and future. She felt that the king's ideas about renunciation were mistaken, but she knew that mere reasoning would not make him understand. He would understand only according to the state of his mind. Therefore she agreed to let him go.

Queen Chudala was perfectly capable of ruling the kingdom fearlessly; indeed, for anyone who has been blessed by Chiti and in whom spiritual wisdom has arisen, the business of running a kingdom would be an ordinary matter. The *Pratyabhijnahridayam* says: *balalābhe viśvaṁ ātmasātkaroti*—"He who has acquired the strength of Chiti can assimilate the universe into himself." Since the whole universe consists of the vibration of Chiti and Chiti had come to live in her heart, there was nothing intimidating about ruling the kingdom. She knew the world as an assemblage of rays of Chiti and the same as her own Self. As a result, she conducted the affairs of state faultlessly and in the best possible way.

The king went off to live in solitude. He found a cave in a forest in the Himalayas, built himself a hut, and started his divine *sadhana* of meditation, concentration, mantra repetition, and asceticism. However, the stricter the disciplines he set himself, the more restless he became, and the more uncontrolled and unsteady his mind. Here, Muktananda says that man can find happiness by living in accordance with his station and upbringing. If he goes against this, then he will find suffering even in happiness. For example, I once had some beautiful and entrancing calves at the Ashram, and out of love for them, I used to feed them all sorts of fruits and sweets which were brought as offerings. As a result, these grass-eating creatures began to get sick. Every creature finds happiness within its own eating and living habits. This was naturally true of the king. For most of his life he had enjoyed the luxury and opulence of a king. Now he was dressed in bark, living in a straw hut, sleeping on a deerskin, and bathing in cold water. He was eating roots and fruits and practicing austerities. As a result, his mind became more and more disturbed, and the more disturbed it got, the more restless he became. He was experiencing, more and more intensely, agitation instead of peace, disharmony instead of equanimity, and melancholy instead of bliss. However, since he was a true seeker he persevered. He thought about renunciation all the time and about what he should give up next. He would think: "*tyāgāchchhāntiranantaram*—'Peace follows renunciation'—and since I haven't found peace it must mean that my renunciation is not yet complete."

His queen, Chudala, was a great yogini. Through the Chiti Shakti she had attained omniscience, and her yoga was so powerful that she could travel wherever she wanted in the Blue Pearl and assume any body she chose. For a long time she had understood her husband's inner state, but she had not been able to impart any of her wisdom to him since he thought of her simply as his wife. She knew she had to wait for the right moment to explain things; if the time was not right, her advice would not be effective. So she refrained and waited in peace. However, through her meditation, she knew everything that happened to the king, everything he did and did not do.

Meanwhile the king went on renouncing more and more. He now only ate fruit—initially every two days, then every three days, then every five days—and his body had begun to shrivel up. It made the queen very unhappy to see him like this, and one day she could contain herself no longer. She changed her body through her yogic power and, taking the form and name of the sage Kumbha, appeared before the king. At the sight of this unknown sage, the king was struck with wonder. He bowed to the sage and arranged for him a place to sit. The sage asked the king how he was, and the king told him everything that was happening inside him. At the end of it all, he said, "O sage, I haven't found peace yet. Can you show me a way?"

Kumbha replied, "King, there is only one mantra: *tyāgāchchhāntiranantaram*—'Peace follows renunciation.'" And with this he disappeared.

When he heard the sage telling him that peace follows renunciation, the king was more astounded than ever. He thought, "I don't understand. What is there left to renounce? I have given up everything, starting with my throne. I gave up riches, property, power, glory, happiness. I gave up my attachment to my family and friends. I live in a grass hut in a mountain cave. And yet this sage comes to me, tells me peace follows renunciation, and vanishes. What else can I give up?" Because the king had not understood the real meaning of renunciation, he had not renounced what he should have, and had renounced what he shouldn't have.

Full of confusion, the king started to think about renunciation all over again. He decided that he would now give up his hut, his deerskin, his water pot, and his bark cloth, and this he did. After he had done this, Kumbha appeared to him once more and said, "O king, are you happy? Have you found peace?"

The king replied, "O sage, I am still trying to find peace. I am desperate."

Kumbha replied, "Your renunciation is not yet complete. Peace follows renunciation." As he said this mantra, he went away, and the king was again left wondering what he could renounce.

Muktananda says that the knowledge of renunciation and acceptance is very complicated. It is a great problem. I always remember something a saint said on the subject:

sāṅḍīmāṅḍi karūṁ jāsī toṁ toṁ vikārā pāvasī nijarūpīṁ bhinna paḍasī
When you give up some things and accept and arrange others,
you fall prey to the wanderings of your mind, and you are
separated from your original Self.

The verses I give below, by Brahmananda, have something interesting
to say about this, and Siddha students can derive much from them:

> O *sadhu*, this is my knowledge, this is my knowledge.
> Both the inert and the conscious in the world have the cons-
> scious as their root and support.
> The whole world has arisen from Consciousness, it is not
> distinct from Consciousness.
> The individual soul is an indestructible part of God—it knows
> no difference or variation.
> One thing is seen in the ocean and a drop, in the sun and in
> a lamp.
> In animal, bird, man, in all life is the boundless, perfect
> Brahman.
> The worldly differences of high and low have been wiped out;
> 'Everything is equal' is the conviction.
> There is no duty of renunciation or acceptance, all doubts
> have been removed.
> The whole expansion of this world manifests as *brahmananda*,
> the bliss of God.

This is how it is. The king should have understood the nature of
renunciation and acceptance, but he was unable to. While a man is
without the full grace of the Guru, when his inner Shakti has not expanded and he has not acquired the power of wisdom through the
blessing of Chiti, he will just renounce and accept whatever he feels
like. It will be completely arbitrary. Until he has acquired the eye
of wisdom he will not be able to look closely into the reality of things,
to recognize renunciation or understand acceptance.

King Shikhidhvaja's renunciation now became even more extreme.
He resolved to renounce everything he possessed, including his life.
He thought, "I'll make a big pyre, burn everything, and then jump
into it myself. When my body is burned, I must find peace." So he
collected dry wood from the forest and piled it up and set it aflame,
and then he took his possessions one by one and, remembering their
associations for him, threw them into the fire. He said to his hut,
"O my hut. I lived in you a long time, but I didn't find peace. Now
I offer you to the fire." To his water pot he said, "O beloved *kaman-
dalu*, I drank water from you for a long time, but I didn't find peace.

Now I give you to the fire." Then he threw his deerskin on the fire, and then taking off his loin cloth, he threw that in too. Now only his naked body was left. He walked round the fire three times and then spoke to his body, "O my dear body, I fed you the six different kinds of flavors until I got tired of satisfying you, but still I found no happiness in you. I bathed you with perfumed oils and waters, but I couldn't find any peace in you. I gave you many girls to enjoy, but still I couldn't find any delight. I washed you, fed you, and adorned you, but I never found any peace." The king was about to leap into the flames when the sage Kumbha again appeared and, grabbing the king's arm, cried, "King, stop, stop! What is this terrible injustice you are about to commit? What is this horrible thing you are going to do?"

"O sage," the king replied, "I've given up everything I own except my body, and still I haven't found peace; so now I am giving it up to the flames. This way I must find peace!"

To this the sage said, "O king! If it is possible to find peace by burning your body in a fire, why haven't all the countless beings that have already died found peace? Is death the way to peace? You are going to burn the body in which you desire the peace and happiness of *jivanmukti*. How can you find peace in the body when you have burned the body? When your body is nothing but ashes, who will enjoy the peace and where will he enjoy it? O king! You don't know what to renounce. Look! In this body, which you can touch and see, there are 72,000 *nadis*, four states of consciousness, four bodies, and five sheaths. Its inner structure is marvelously framed. It came from the union of your father's sperm and your mother's ovum. Half of it you owe to your father's sperm and the other half to your mother's ovum, and both halves are united in one body. In this body, what is yours to renounce?

"O king, the sexual fluids of your parents were formed from the food they ate. And that came from the earth. What is there that you have the right to renounce? Man eats the food growing in the earth, spends his life on the earth's surface and finally merges with the earth. The body is pervaded by the earth, and into this body the supremely peaceful Lord enters in the form of the Self—and the Self is not yours either. Your physical sense organs—the eye, ear, nose, tongue, and skin—are not yours, for the different deities enter them and make them perform their different functions. King, you are going to give up this body. What is your renunciation in all this? Furthermore, just as your body is pervaded by earth because it is born on the earth, lives on the earth, and is absorbed into the earth, so the earth is pervaded by water because it is born from water. Water is pervaded by fire because it is born from fire, and fire is pervaded by air, and air is pervaded by ether, and ether is pervaded by God. In all this there is nothing that is yours. It is only the illusion of "mine" in all this that you have to recognize and renounce. You were going to renounce a body that someone else had given you, believing it to be your own renunciation. The truth is that when through the grace of the Guru you have acquired the eye of wisdom, there is nothing to renounce except this illusion."

> *ito na kinchit parato na kinchit*
> *yato yato yāmi tato na kinchit*
> *vichārya paśyāmi jaganna kinchit*
> *svātmāvabodhāt adhikaṁ na kinchit*

There is nothing here, nothing there,
Wherever I go there is nothing.
When I contemplate, I see that the world is nothing,
There is nothing more than the realization of my own Self.

The king saw that what the sage said was perfectly true. The body to which he had turned hostile was really his helper. The body was a means and not an obstruction. I remember a verse on this theme:

> *sādhaka jaga heṁ bādhā nāhī yā pāsuni tuja leśa*
> *tujalā yāchā dveṣa kāṁ re*

This world is helpful; it is not even a little bit obstructive. Why do you hate it?

What kind of renunciation is it to renounce the body through which we experience the fruits of good and bad *karma*, to despise it and ruin its health through living in the wrong way? What kind of renunciation is it to debilitate the body in which you have to live for a long time, through lack of discipline and self-control? You have to use your brains when it comes to renunciation. What you have to renounce is the root of all suffering, that highly dangerous thing called *abhinivesha*. This is defined in the scriptures: to regard something as ours which does not belong to us, or to identify ourselves with that which is not the Self. This ego is the cause of all our afflictions. It has reduced God to a limited individual soul, turned happiness into sorrow and transformed the One into the many. If *aham*, the individual ego, is destroyed and replaced by *So'ham*, "I am He," what is left to renounce? The whole world is filled with Chiti. If your renunciation is purposeless or goes against the scriptures, you will get confusion instead of peace. The poet-saint Banarasi has written on this theme:

Ram is not attained by renouncing wealth or life;
Only he attains Narayana who renounces the pride of his body.

God can never be attained by renouncing all worldly affairs,
By renouncing wife, children, family, or household matters,
By eating only roots, tubers, and fruit, and renouncing
   other foods,
By renouncing clothes and going about naked, by giving up
   women,
Even by renouncing one's own life force, Hari is not attained.

Ram is not attained by renouncing wealth or life;
Only he attains Narayana who renounces the pride of his body.

By renouncing beds of flowers, diamonds, and pearls,
By renouncing one's own caste and family traditions,
By renouncing the entanglements of this world and roaming
   through the forest day and night,
By renouncing remembrance of the body and burning it
   to ashes,
By renouncing one's own life, without any knowledge of
   Brahman;

Ram is not attained by renouncing wealth or life;
Only he attains Narayana who renounces the pride of his body.

By renouncing all speech, by observing silence and saying
   nothing,
By renouncing father and grandfather and practicing yoga
   from childhood,

By renouncing one's own good mother, one's tuft of hair and
sacred thread,
By renouncing killing and violence and never harming any
living creature,
If the pride of the body is not abandoned, what can be
attained by renouncing all these things?

Ram is not attained by renouncing wealth or life;
Only he attains Narayana who renounces the pride of his body.

By renouncing the bed of earth, by not sleeping but standing
day and night,
By renouncing all ease, doing without comforts, and undergoing hardship,
By renouncing bitter words and speaking sweetly to all,
By renouncing all these things but not abandoning the constant pride of the body,
Banarasi says, even after renouncing all life, still He is not
attained.

Ram is not attained by renouncing wealth or life;
Only he attains Narayana who renounces the pride of his body.

This is an authoritative poem for Siddha students. Actually, undis-
criminating renunciation is the most binding enjoyment, whereas
discriminating enjoyment is the highest renunciation. Why did God
create this phenomenal universe from his own harmonious magnitude?
What was the reason? For whom and for what was this world created?
If a Siddha student doesn't think about these things and just takes
to nonscriptural renunciation, he is unworthy. It is because human
society does not have a true understanding of the world that it is so
unhappy, but if the world could be properly understood, could be
seen as the play of Chiti, then our entire life would become divine.
Since this world, created by God, is identical with the Self, it is thus
the very form of Paramatman, the supreme Self. It is a principle of
Vedantic philosophy that the effect is no different from the cause,
that cause is inherent in effect.

In some scriptures it is said that the world is unreal, and without
joy, and that it is an obstacle. If a seeker, out of a spiritual impulse,
devotes himself a little to the search for God, he is repeatedly told

that the world is false, transient, and joyless. He starts believing it to be true. These concepts are very harmful, since the world becomes as you see it. In India some mothers stop their children's crying by telling them that there is a ghost in the house which will catch them if they don't be quiet. This ghost, which remains in the child's mind for a long time, is created by the mother for the child. Westerners do not have such fears, for they do not give their children such false terrors. In the same way, the writers of some scriptures have for some reason described the world as unreal, harsh, empty, and futile, but it is in fact not so. Who else except Chiti has the power to become so many worlds? The world is nothing but the sport of Chiti, who abounds in infinite forms.

To live in a world filled with Chiti without seeing and understanding that Chiti exists equally everywhere is the opposite of true knowledge. However, it is true that as long as man himself is false, dry, and empty, the world will also appear to be the same. This is self-evident—as you yourself are, so the world is. Whether you are a householder, an ascetic, a monk, or a mendicant, the world reflects your own state. To one who has received the Guru's grace, whose inner Shakti is awakened, and who has seen the play of Chiti in his heart, the outside world is the blossoming of Chiti. He sees the pulsations of Chiti everywhere. I am again reminded of this mantra:

> *śrīgurucharaṇāmbhojaṁ   satyameva   vijānatām*
> *jagat satyamasatyaṁ vā netareti matirmama*

To one who knows the Guru's feet as the sole reality it does not matter whether the world is real or unreal.

Whether the world is real or not is no longer important to that person. The reality or unreality of the world is nothing but a debate, from which you don't obtain anything. When the mind frees itself from these controversies the play of Chiti can be perceived, and in such a condition the world appears as God. A man who has attained realization sees the Lord in the world—not emptiness or joylessness. The ideas that arise during *sadhana* are discovered to be inauthentic in the state of realization. It is like the division in scriptures between pre-revelation and post-revelation. Pre-revelation is weak, whereas

post-revelation is strong. Pre-revelation states: *aputrasya gatirnāsti—*
"A man who has no son is not liberated after death." The question
should then be asked, "Should a renunciant get married?" And how
was it possible for celibates like Narada, Sanatakumara, and others to
attain liberation? However, post-revelation states: *na karmaṇā na
prajayā dhanena tyāgenaike amritatvamānaśuḥ (Mahanarayana Upanishad* 8:14)—"Immortality comes not from good deeds or a son or
wealth; immortality can be attained only through renunciation."

It is not renunciation of home, family, responsibilities, food,
nor of the body or of selfless action that is implied by this, but the
renunciation of differentiation, of our *abhinivesha.* As soon as we
renounce this "I," the truth lying hidden within us is revealed, and
the truth lying hidden in the phenomenal world is also revealed. One
Chiti can be seen flowing through all the sense organs and all their
objects. Man's weeping ceases forever. He begins to carry out his
worldly affairs with ease and reverence, seeing God underlying them all.

It was like this with Queen Chudala. She was a perfect yogini
who had realized Brahman, who was a devoted and virtuous wife,
and to whom the play of Chiti was absolutely real. She saw the universe as the outward vibration of Chiti. She had her cave of equanimity
right in her own palace and was always aware of the presence of God
in whatever she was doing. Since she had renounced the sense of
differentiation and saw that all things were the vibrations of Chiti,
her renunciation was perfect, in the scriptural sense. She had not
renounced her home but the tendency to differentiate, which separates
one from one's true Self. Thus she was as free from anxiety in day-
to-day affairs as she was peaceful in meditation. For her:

> *viṣayeṣu cha sarveṣu indriyārtheṣu cha sthitam*
> *yatra yatra nirūpyeta nāśivaṁ vidyate kvachit*

Whatever is observed, in all objects and in all sense impressions, nothing inauspicious is found anywhere.

That is, Queen Chudala had reached the state in which she could see
Chiti pulsating in all objects, in all sense impressions. Never at any
time did she see anything other than Shiva. So, always seeing the
divine in the world, Chudala spent her time filled with God.

After he had been instructed by the sage Kumbha, King Shikhidhvaja completely renounced his wrong identification. His mind, which had hitherto flowed outward, immediately turned inward. As it went deeper and deeper, it assumed the form of the Self and then became the Self. The king passed into a deep *samadhi* in which he was aware only of oneness. He transcended the distinctions of inner and outer, of duality and category, and found peace. He was like an insomniac who falls at last into a long sleep, lying by a cool and pleasant water spring and fanned by soft winds. When it at last finds peace, a mind which has been constantly restless gives up its mind-ness and becomes one with the Self. King Shikhidhvaja, having attained his desire, became absorbed in his inner happiness. When he emerged from this state of bliss and became aware of the external world, he experienced the same happiness there too. What he had experienced within was revealed outside. The sense of differentiation had vanished completely from his heart. Outside he saw what he had discovered within.

The king now really understood the principle: *yathā atra tathā anyatra*—"As here, so elsewhere." His viewpoint had changed. He renounced his wrong understanding about renunciation. He put aside multiplicity and embraced unity; he renounced his false renunciation and awoke to the reality of his own Self. This vision of undifferentiated unity destroyed multiplicity for him. Seeing the One in all, he wiped away his foolish ideas of duality. He began to see the Lord of the universe everywhere; he saw His radiance in slums and cremation grounds, in gardens and groves of trees, in fruits and flowers. He saw the division between solitude and society as the play of delusion. He saw that distinctions like "This is a forest, this is an uninhabited land, this place is full of people, this is a place for workers to live" were unreal. The veil of distinction was burned away in the fire of knowledge. He realized that whatever could be found in a forest, in a cave, or in solitude could be found in his own palace. When he knew this with certainty, he wanted to go back to his own palace, and he set off for home.

It will perhaps surprise Siddha students that such a great renunciant should go back home. Dear students! Things like acceptance and renunciation, high and low, have meaning only as long as you have not found realization. When you are realized, what is different from you? Everything is your own beauty.

The unenlightened and the enlightened have one thing in common: they both have to bear the consequences of their past actions. While the unenlightened man is always subjugated to the differentiating mentality and suffers these consequences weeping and wailing and complaining, the enlightened man sees the world as a play of Chiti and bears the consequences of his actions with the knowledge that the world is the light of his Self. Both the ignorant and the enlightened must live their lives, but one experiences life in terms of outward sense objects, whereas for the other it is the divine play of Chiti.

The enlightened man, since he has the merit accumulated through countless births, will go through life supported by beauty and material wealth, but in spite of these things he will not be born again, and he will not be trapped in worldly enjoyments. A yogi like this lives ecstatically, turning sensuous enjoyment into pure yoga. He finds his delight in the Self, not in the senses. To worldly people he appears worldly, but his state is that of a great yogi absorbed in the Absolute. For him, the whole of empirical existence is the supreme Reality. This constant awareness of the Absolute is his meditation. Thus, his meditation cannot be interrupted even when he is busy in the world.

For ordinary people sense enjoyment is one thing and the goal of meditation another. The ordinary meditator has to direct his mind toward the spiritual goal in order to drive out his craving for enjoyment. But for the great yogi absorbed in Brahman everything is meditation, because all his actions are filled with Parabrahman. His daily bathing, eating, drinking, coming and going, and wearing of clothes and ornaments are all meditation. I call this incessant meditation, which continues day and night. In Tukaram's words it is *viṣaya to jyāmchā jhālā nārāyaṇa*—"It is a meditation in which all material pleasures have become God."

Through the inspiration of Chiti Shakti, all states and modes of being can come to such a Siddha yogi. Depending on his destiny, he may become a king and live in grandeur and magnificence or he may be withdrawn like Jadabharat, or a naked *avadhuta* like Rishabhadeva; his behavior may be stupid, intoxicated, or demoniacal. Chiti, who enters within us and fills us with Shiva, may bring us honor or disgrace, riches or hardship; these are all gifts of Her grace. Since these conditions are all determined by Shiva, we will experience His love in them. But I am speaking only for those men and women who have received the grace of the Guru. Those who are not thus blessed find suffering even in happiness.

Once he had received the grace of the Guru and the knowledge that the universe is pervaded by Chiti, King Shikhidhvaja saw that his throne, his subjects, his wife, and his relatives were all filled with the play of Chiti, and that they were aids to happiness and full of happiness. Now he found the highest joy in the things that had once driven him wild with pain. He accepted the position given him by his destiny and passed his days ruling his kingdom. He saw Jagadish, the Lord of the universe, in the heat of the sun, in mountain peaks, in the courses of flowing rivers, in the jumping waves of the ocean, in the deluges of the rainy season, in the lightning of the clouds, in fields of yellow, green, and blue, and in the immense spaces of the skies. He experienced the pulsations of Chiti in hunger and thirst, hope and despair, nearness and distance, justice and injustice, greed and contentment, anger and agitation. In spite of seeing differences in the outside world, inwardly he experienced nondifferentiation. He had fully realized the Truth. He saw the light of his inner Self in his carriages, his jewelry, his food and drink, in god, man, seer and sage, in wood and in stone. He would find God in all the names, forms, qualities, and principles of the moving and unmoving universe.

In fact it is our tendency to differentiate that is the root cause of man's fear and lack of peace. The *Brihadaranyaka Upanishad* says of those who are subject to differentiation: *mrityoh sa mrityumāpnoti ya iha nāneva paśyati* (IV:4:19)—"He who sees objects as different from one another goes from death to death." The *Taittiriya Upanishad* says: *udaramantaram kurūte'th tasya bhayam bhavati* (2:7)—"If one perceives even the slightest difference, one is subject to fear." Truth, the consciousness of equality in all things, the awareness of the Self in all, and firm faith in the Guru's wisdom constitute the best path to fearlessness.

Just as a fish can be thirsty even in the ocean, a man bereft of Guru's grace will see this blissful world as dead, dreary, and empty.

This ignorant individual imagines a snake in a piece of rope and starts to sweat and shake with fear. In the same way, he projects imperfections onto the world. He sees the world which is like a sheaf of radiating beams of Chiti, as material, as barren, as *maya*, and suffers intolerably. This is mainly because he lacks the grace and teaching of a Guru. Man is in such a condition because the inner Shakti has not grown and expanded in him. Vasuguptacharya says of man in this state: *śaktidaridraḥ saṁsārī*—"One bereft of Shakti is a transmigratory soul."

If all men, women, boys, and girls win the grace of a Guru and have their inner Shakti awakened, then all these people, while still living in the world, will see the concentration of Chiti revealed in the heart. *Svaśaktivikāse tu śiva eva*—"When his own Shakti is awakened, the individual soul becomes supreme Shiva." He belongs to Shiva; he is in Shiva; he is Shiva. Muktananda says: When you win the grace of the Guru, you will become Shiva in no time.

All men and women can meditate, for they are identical images of God. Just as meditation brings the spiritual journey of yogis to consummation, so it brings the mundane journey of worldly people to consummation. In meditation the power of memory increases. Many of the boys and girls who come to Shree Gurudev Ashram used to be poor students, but through the wonderful influence of meditation, they have passed their exams with the highest marks. When in your meditation the mind becomes steady, the *prana* becomes very pure. Physical torpor is then destroyed and enthusiasm and energy are increased. Enthusiasm and energy are very helpful friends in the world. Through meditation the *nadis* are purified and many sicknesses destroyed. Indeed, many of the students of meditation who come to the Ashram have completely conquered disease. Furthermore, through the inner realizations of meditation, a divinely inspired mutual respect grows between husbands and wives. Brothers and sisters see the divine in each other and the relationships between children, parents, and in-laws are filled with a divine emotion. This is known as *svargamay samsar*—"life filled with heaven." This is the fruit of the yoga of meditation.

O you who live in the world! No matter what happens you always set aside time to eat, and you should also find time to meditate.

Whenever you get the time, sit peacefully, let your mind steady itself in the heart, pray to Sri Gurudev, and meditate. Keep on singing the great mantra that the Guru gave you, whatever you are doing. If you don't get time to meditate during the day, meditate while you are going to sleep. This way you will certainly find happiness. Whenever you get a little time to yourself, make the best of it and meditate.

I also give you a mantra from the text *Jnanarnava* which a Siddha student can reflect on even when he is not meditating.

> *aham na nārako nāma na tiryag nāpi mānuṣaḥ*
> *na devaḥ kintu siddhātma sarvo 'yam karmavikramaḥ*

If we contemplate ourselves, we will see that we are not demons or animals or men or gods; we are simply the essence of perfection, perfect souls.

Repeat this over and over again until you really understand it, until it is fixed in your mind.

King Janaka became realized while living in the world. Take to heart this piece of wisdom, which he told his queen:

> *bheda bhāvanā taja de sumate*
> *sarva mem ātmabuddhi kara le*
> *putra vāsanā loka vāsanā deha vāsanā taja de*

O wise men! Give up the idea of diversity and see the Self in everything. Give up attachment to children, to society, and to the body.

For the sake of renunciation, King Janaka once turned away from the world. For a period he gave up food and drink and no longer ruled his kingdom. However, his renunciation quickly led him to complete knowledge of oneness; indeed, if renunciation does not lead to this, it has been a fake. As soon as he attained knowledge of the equality of all and understood the identity of the Self with the whole world, he became satisfied and returned to rule his kingdom. Outwardly he watched over the affairs of state, and inwardly he experienced the presence of God. Janaka's queen, seeing how peaceful and serene and loving he had become in his heart, became curious and asked him how to find peace. The king replied, "O queen, the whole world is the Self.

When this knowledge reveals itself from within, the whole universe, animate and inanimate, is seen as the light of the Self. O goddess, there are then no distinctions such as individual, world, mind, *maya,* and thought. Outside and inside, in yourself and in others, you perceive only one Chiti. O goddess, the feeling of difference that exists in the Self as the world is the state of a bound soul. And differentiation is the reason for suffering. You can never find peace in this condition. The more you attempt to escape the world by practicing mantra repetition and asceticism, the more you thrust yourself into it. O queen, I am not an individual being, I am the Self. All this is my creative energy—outside, inside, above, below. There is nothing other than me. In this world, that which appears inert and that which appears conscious is not separate from me. This wisdom, this insight that I am giving you, brings the greatest peace. It is the ocean of boundless joy."

In fact, the mind becomes active when it exists separately from the Self. It is this activity of the mind, separate from the Self, which creates *samsara,* worldly involvement and bondage. When you see your own Self vibrating in the moving and unmoving universe, the mind—*chitta*—ceases its activity and becomes Chiti. When the mind of a Siddha student has become Chiti, he becomes the king of the empire of Chiti. He sees the Self everywhere. Then body, *maya,* differentiation, and duality are all lost in nonduality. The pure One, the goal described by the authors of the scriptures as Satchidananda, Being-Consciousness-Bliss, appears in all names and forms. This world is as one sees it. When the light of the Self shines in the eyes, the whole cosmos can be seen vibrating in the form of the Self. When the sun rises, darkness turns into light. In the same way, when knowledge of the Self dawns, the world appears as the Self. Differentiation is at the root of all misery. Differentiation has made many suffer by making them dance in duality. Differences are not real, but appear to be so. By the Guru's grace the curtain of differentiation and duality is drawn aside, and when the seeker receives this grace, he finds Godhood within himself. This is *jivanmukti,* the state of liberation while living in the body.

Jivanmukti is the attainment of *sahajavastha,* the state of pure and natural spontaneity. This is the best state for a man to attain.

The *sadhana* of love is a very high *sadhana.* Love is also called *bhakti,* or devotion. Love is a dynamic and inspiring throbbing of the heart. Love is the very nature of God, whom the scriptural authors have called supreme Bliss, and Satchidananda. It exists in its fullness within man. Even if he does not experience it, it is nonetheless there. A blind man who has never seen the light may say when he hears others talk about it, "There is no light. I have never seen it. I don't know anything about it." Yet the light exists; it is only that he has no eyes. Similarly there is love, whether or not it is experienced. If you have not followed the path of love, if you have not tried to find it, how can it be attained?

Love is nectar. Love is immortal. Through love alone, the *gopis* of Gokul found God. Love is a glimpse of the secret inner cave. Love that dwells within flows out through the different sense organs. When it flows to the eyes, it makes forms beautiful; when it flows to the ears, it makes sounds melodious; when it rises to the tongue, it makes tastes sweet and pleasing. Love is the blissful Self whose outward expression makes sensuous objects enjoyable. If this outpouring throb of love were to stop, the senses would become lifeless, joyless, useless, just as zeros without a digit in front are meaningless, and nothing but zeros.

In your ordinary life, learn to love. This love should be pure, unattached, and given for its own sake. If it contains any demands, it is just a commercial exchange—the motions of love, but not love itself. Real love contains no demands, no "mine and yours," no selfishness.

Love is just love.   Sri Guru Nityananda is that love.   Just love the Sadguru.   Don't ask him even for liberation.   There is enough love in the human heart for not just one man but for thousands, but because of desire and useless thinking, an unfortunate person cannot see it. Once he becomes free of these, he discovers pure, immortal, and complete love.

To find love you must first of all love yourself.   Do not torture yourself by repeating that you are impure, joyless, unreal, ephemeral, or miserable.   Certain religions, certain communities, certain poetic works consider the body vile, weak, and petty, with no more worth than a shell.   How unjust!   Tukaram says, *Brahmabhūta hote kāyā cha kīrtanī*–"Through repeating God's name the body becomes divine." How unfairly you treat the body that becomes divine through remembrance of God, meditation, devoted worship, and love for the Guru!

I have seen many *sadhakas* treating their bodies harshly, and as a result, all that they eventually attain is some disease.

O Siddha students!   Your live body is the temple of Goddess Chiti. Treat it with respect by being pure and chaste, by eating good, wholesome food, and by wearing beautiful, simple, clean clothes.

O Siddha students!   If others call this body low, let them.   You should not forget that salvation is attained through this very body.   If you want to attain your beloved God and Guru and unfold the inner source of love, you must first love yourself.   Only love will take you to God.   You desire inner peace, but hate your body and senses.   You long for inner joy, but are as hostile to the body, which is a means to that joy, as if it were your worst enemy.   First, fully know your body. Once you know your inner being, you will realize that the body is not illusory but a beautiful temple filled with knowledge; by loving it you will make your own spring of love flow.

Understand that the ever-new joy that reveals itself in meditation dwells in the heart as a free, inspiring force.   Develop this love, and let it flow from you to others.

Love should not be for the satisfaction of the senses or for selfish ends, for then it is just attachment and not love of God; attachment is impure and can never bring you to God.   Love increases through giving, not through taking.   The feeling of "mine and yours" is a great obstacle in love.   Your love should be equal and unparalleled.

Dear Siddha students! If you want to find love, you must have a true understanding of the body, the dwelling place of love. You must have knowledge of the functions of its five component elements. Your attitude toward your body should be pure, friendly, respectful, and affectionate. The body has been man's companion and friend through many births, through many different journeys of pain and happiness. The body is a fundamental necessity of *sadhana*. It is the ladder to the city of liberation; it is the great temple of the inner Self. In the innermost part of this bodily temple, God, the Lord of love, lives as the inner Self. Muktananda therefore says that, when a Siddha student achieves understanding of the body and sees that it is the temple of the inner Self, he will never do anything unfriendly to it nor involve it in anything degrading nor defile it through depraved or immoral acts.

Some people regard the body as a place of pleasure, like a club or a hotel or a cinema, and thus destroy its purity and lose their Shakti. In my opinion, they insult their bodies instead of honoring them and treating them justly. There are also some disturbed people who torture and repress their pure and friendly bodies in a way that is cruel and unnatural. Their hearts, which should be filled with love, are filled with lamentation. They hurt their bodies day and night. They constantly pray to the Lord to free them from the prison of the body. But the truth is that your body is without fault.

The body is made of five elements and is the home of your Self. It is a land where you experience joy and sorrow. The body is the servant of the Self. It is always at your service and ready to go wherever you take it. If you want to take it to hell, it will go there as soon as you ask it. If you want to take it to heaven, it will willingly go there. If you seat it on an elephant or a horse, it's happy. If you feed it *khir*, *puris*, and *halva*, it's happy; if you feed it chilies, chutney, and dry bread, it's happy too. It's happy with everything. It's happy if you adorn it with jewels, but it's just as pleased with torn old clothes or a loin cloth. The body is such a servant, such a slave, such a friend that there is no one else in the world like it.

There was once a devoted servant of the Guru. One day someone asked this man, "How are you feeling? Tell me about your joys and your sorrows. What is your life in the ashram like? How do the heat and cold affect you?"

The man replied, "Sir, I know nothing about the heat of summer or the cold of winter, I am a servant. I only know how to serve. My Guru alone knows about my cold, my heat, my joys, and my sufferings." How wonderful! This man had completely lost himself in his service to the Guru; he had kept nothing back for himself. This is how love should be. It should always be free from defect, differentiation, anguish, and desire. Love like this will lead you to God and will make you God.

Think of the five primal elements that make up your body. Think of earth, which is so beautiful, which is the womb of many different kinds of food and the mother of so many different beings. Think of pure water, which brings life to grains, flowers, fruit, trees, and plants, which is so full of love that it washes everything of its dirt and is the friend of everyone. How full of love it is! Think of fire, which lives in all beings according to their needs and is equally the friend of all. In man it becomes the gastric fire and digests food. It lives in wood, in stone, and in every object in keeping with the nature of each. It is a wonderful example of all-pervading, desireless love. Think of air, which is the life of man, his *prana*. It pervades everything in the world, animate and inanimate, in equal measure. It sustains the movement of the universe and everything in it. Once *prana* leaves the body, it becomes a useless corpse. Think finally of ether, which reminds us of the detachment of the inner Self and which encompasses all activities in its vast spaces. These are the five elements of which the body is composed, and the conscious Self pervades every cell. First, contemplate fully this beautiful and desireless body, and then love it as God.

Think about it. If your eyes see someone else's wealth or beauty and burn with anger, greed, and envy, isn't it madness to get angry with them and damage them or put them out? Is it proper to punish your innocent eyes in the name of renunciation and asceticism? They are your steadfast friends. Your eyes are not attracted to anything or repulsed by anything; they are simply friends who help you see forms. No matter how you make use of your senses, they are only helpful to you. They are prepared to do whatever work you give them. If you want to become a yogi of love in the body, they are willing; if you want to be angry, they are willing. Whatever you become, your body will become. Whatever you want to express, that's what it becomes.

Understand your body properly. Without desire, love the sun and moon seated in your eyes, the deities seated in all your senses, the different parts of the body such as the hands and feet. Then discover and worship the Lord beyond quality who dwells in the qualities of the senses. Worship with deep and desireless love, not mechanically. You must practice restraint; the senses must be controlled. But do not torture the body or make it sick in the name of restraint and renunciation.

You should get to know the various powers that live in your body —in the sense organs, muscles, nerves, and brain. They are not antagonistic to you. They are neither auspicious for you nor are they inauspicious. They are neither good nor are they bad. They are absolutely detached. They act according to the mind and the inner tendencies. Man's inner Shakti is God's Shakti. The same divine Shakti assumes at different times the forms of desire, anger, infatuation, greed, and so on, and uses one or another of the sense organs as Her vehicle. Muktananda says: Meditate. Make love come alive. As love begins to pulsate in all the senses, natural renunciation, natural yoga, and natural knowledge will arise within you. It is because your mind does not see any love in itself that it looks for it in others, that it searches for love through the senses and for objects of enjoyment in the outside world. If man were to see and love himself as God, why would he look outside? What is outside anyway? Love comes in meditation.

The indulgent man will go on satisfying his senses until his body becomes useless. In the end his worn-out body torments him, and he begins to hate it. The renunciant too wears out his body with his unnatural forms of austerity. He develops enmity toward the body and tortures it, making it useless, yet desires the happiness of liberation. First understand your body, which is the vehicle for your journey toward liberation, maintain it carefully, and then look on it with love and respect.

Your body is a marvelous work of art created by God, a beautiful storehouse full of intelligence, a mine of secret knowledge. To enter the court of God, to journey to Vaikuntha, to see Kailasa, or to roam in the city of stillness, you are going to use the body. What will you do if you abandon it? Knowledge of the Self arises in the body, through meditation. Truly, Muktananda, isn't it madness if, after attaining this divine and priceless body, you constantly fight with it instead of transcending it? What sort of renunciation is it to hate this body instead of loving it?

Man has acquired a body through the compassion of God. If instead of becoming a lover of inner and outer existence and getting drunk on the nectar of those endless love-rays scattered throughout the *sahasrara,* he offers his body the poisonous, polluted, and deadly drink of sensual indulgence, then isn't he the king of the insane? Do not dry up the bodily fluids, but increase them through love. It is this that will bring you to union with God.

I once read an authentic account of the death of a saint who was a man of knowledge and was always absorbed in meditation. He had fore-knowledge of his death, and when the time came, he gathered everyone around him, asked them for their blessings and forgiveness, and then thanked them. After that, he bowed to the four directions, to the five elements, and to his Guru, the giver of wisdom. Last of all he thanked and honored his body, the walking, moving, speaking temple of God, given by God, in which he had completed his spiritual journey and had seen God. With folded hands he addressed his body: "My beloved body, by your grace and help I have reached God. I thank you. I have often inconvenienced and frightened you. I have made you go through so much anguish and torment on my behalf. But no matter what I did you always helped me. Truly I am in your debt. O my dear body! You endowed me with a quick and perceptive mind. Through you I attained the *nirvikalpa* state in meditation, the highest state of all. So my dear friend, I shall always be indebted to you. Knowingly and unknowingly I wronged you many times, but you always helped me and always did everything you could for me. Whatever I did to you, you never gave me anything but your friendship and your companionship in return. But for you I could not have done good *sadhana* and could not have reached God." Having said this to the body, the saint merged with the Absolute.

Dear Siddha students, you too should have this exalted attitude toward your bodies. Have the same reverent and respectful love. When I read the loving words that saint addressed to his body, I feel a tremendous joy beating in my heart. If you could listen to them the way I do, you would soon be filled with the highest bliss. I ask, my dear Siddha students, did you ever look on your body with such desireless love?

Did you ever love it with pure Self-contemplation, with meditation, hymns and chanting, with the *So'ham* mantra repeated on your incoming and outgoing breaths? Did you ever thank it by making vows of restraint, by offering it foods which bring long life, giving it sweet and pure juices? If not, how ungrateful you have been! How ill-mannered! What could be worse than treating your dear friend like this! Dear seekers! You should contemplate the body, understand what it is, develop a desireless friendship with it, tend it punctually and regularly. If you really understand your body, you will fill it with yoga, love, and meditation.

It is the mind with its ceaseless thoughts and fancies that takes the body all over the place. The body runs after thoughts and thoughts run after the mind. The mind gives orders to the body and senses. Why do you punish the body in order to please the mind? Why do you punish Krishna when you are angry with Ram? What purpose does it serve? I agree that the mind is fickle and unsteady and causes us trouble. It is only to control the mind that so many techniques have been devised. Yogis learn these techniques to bring their minds under control, but they still become votaries of pride and ego, devotees of easy living. They don't find love through these practices, nor do they find inner contentment or joy in their hearts. Everybody says that the mind never stays in one place, and I entirely agree. But at the same time, have you ever shown it a good place to rest? Take the mind to a worthy place and it will stay there. It won't wander here and there.

There was a swami who lived in a small and simple hut in a village. He did not own much, but lived feeling rich in the midst of poverty. One day the richest merchant in the nearby town decided to visit him, but on arriving discovered that the swami was out. A disciple offered him a place to sit. The merchant did not sit and kept pacing up and down by a tree outside. The disciple was surprised at the merchant's behavior. When the swami got home, the disciple, in astonished tones, recounted what had happened. The swami was not in the least surprised. "Brother," he explained, "we are mendicants, after all. There is no suitable place here for him to sit, so naturally he walked up and down outside." Your mind is like that merchant. Only when it gets a good place will it stop wandering. Beloved brothers! You are in the same condition. Your mind is always trying to get hold of something it really likes, something really good. O mind! You have tried everything, searched everywhere for happiness and peace, for something to engage you, but you are still restless and depressed. Your search for knowledge only made you melancholy. You mastered a branch of yoga and for a while blossomed with life, but then you fell. You searched among sensual pleasures, but didn't find love. You became a worm in the mire of sense pleasures. Still no satisfaction, no stability, only nightmares of anxiety.

You must now learn a new lesson. Love everyone boundlessly, desirelessly, uniquely. If you have never loved anyone, how can you find peace? Brother, you must become pure, unattached, and without that ill will that makes you see differences. There is nothing in God's creation that is against you, that wishes you ill. You should learn to make God's creation friendly to you. If your mind could go deep within yourself even once, it would stay there. Do not consider your mind as an enemy. It has great power, but you will only be able to utilize it if you understand it first. Some yogis are able to show you all sorts of miracles just by ordinary mental power. If you really come to know your mind, you will see what a wonderful worker it is. The mind is a magnificent and creative power.

Contemplate the fickleness of the mind; it is this very unsteadiness of the mind which has attracted you to the great knowledge of Siddha Yoga and which has brought you to Ganeshpuri. The mind is so restless that even when you show it the most beautiful things it cannot enjoy them properly. One day it's interested in beauty, the next day in tastes, the next day in fragrances, the next day in sounds or something else. This restlessness and agitation constantly drives it onward in its search for a fine and good place. If the mind did not fluctuate, an angry person would be angry all the time, a greedy person greedy at every moment, the deluded immersed in their delusions, and the lustful perpetually lustful. The rich would be absorbed only in their riches, the artist only in his art. But it does not happen like that. Everywhere you hear the same mantra, that peace is not in money, art, beauty, sense pleasures, or anything else. Because it is not in these things, the mind wanders from one place to the next and constantly suffers. Finally, the restlessness of the mind makes you desperate.

Muktananda says: Dear students, the mind wants real love, complete equanimity, and union with God. The mind wants something captivating; that is why it is restless. It leaves one place of restlessness and goes on to the next. Just as a bee flies from one flower to another collecting honey, the mind, for one reason or another, wanders on and on. But remember that there is a significant quest behind this restlessness of the mind: the mind is looking for perfect repose. The mind will always fluctuate and will never be steady until it is completely dissolved in meditation on the Self. Only when it has become lost in meditation as a gift of Kundalini and become one with the inner light will it abandon its unsteadiness and become still. Remember that only when the mind becomes completely still in the Self in meditation, and absorbed in love, will you become the incarnation of supreme bliss. Your direction will change; you will be transformed. A fountain of pure peace will flow inside you.

The mind cannot find perfect repose anywhere except in God. When you meet God, you find everything, and the mind becomes steady. Then, even if you try, it doesn't move. From this point of view, it is the restlessness of your mind, that has never been satisfied by temporary stillness, which has set you on the search for truth and peace. The mind does not become still anywhere except in God. It is this tendency of the mind which has led it to find peace. You should consider this a great service on the part of the mind. The restlessness of your mind is a great asset to you, for it has fostered your interest in meditation and has made you worthy of the grace of the Siddhas. So you should welcome heartily the beneficent grace of the mind.

Dear seekers! Remember the words of Muktananda, which are like a mantra and are also filled with his actual experience. No matter with how much pride one may say, "My religion is the best," if the mind does not find repose there, then it is not God's abode. No matter how much one may hear someone praise a mantra saying, "It is a great and true mantra," if the mind does not become happy there, then it is not God's dwelling place. No matter how prominent a sect may be, no matter how great a guru may be—whether he performs wonderful miracles, drinks holy water, applies sacred ash, or worships gods and goddesses—if the mind does not find repose there, then even that is not God's abode. If the mind stops for a moment at a place and then moves on agitatedly, it means there is no peace at that place. You can try and stop the mind, but it will always want to move on. It runs on and on looking for happiness. If you want it to stop, you must plunge it in love, thrust it deep into the love of the Self. Where there is an illusion of peace, the mind will stop momentarily and then, more restless than ever, run on again. But where it is really happy, it stops running and finds repose.

Instead of trying to control and force your mind, you should lead it lovingly to the river of the ecstasy of the Self. Take it on that pilgrimage to the divine shade of the love of the Self, where the luster of true love shines. If you turn the mind to the supremely blissful Self, it will want to run there as fast as it can, but if you stubbornly try to make it peaceful by force or by austerities, it will become more and more agitated and turn against you. Love the mind, but even before you love it, stop thinking of it as the mind. Regard it as the Goddess Chiti who is pulsating as the mind. Give up your antagonism to it and, establishing a true friendship with it, say, "Go to the inner Self." To think like this is actually meditation. If you are going to conquer the mind you must love it, considering that it is filled with Chiti. When you think of the mind as ordinary, when you are hostile to it, then the mind conquers you. Therefore, to conquer the mind completely, you must love it. Love is a mantra of victory. It is the magnet that draws God to you. It is the great *yajna* that makes the mind intoxicated and joyful. Love has great power. It makes the impossible possible; it has the power to make the broken whole. Cease to think of yourselves as small and petty. Fill yourselves with love, and you will see your own greatness.

Dear yogis of meditation! Through meditation you can discover what is inside you and what is not inside you. Without meditation you are poor; with it you are rich. So first love yourself and meditate with love.

There was once a Siddha who lived in a forest. One day he was visited by a seeker who said to him, "Maharaj! I want to see God. What sadhana should I do?"

After studying him carefully the Siddha asked, "Who do you love?"

"Love is an obstacle on the path to God," the seeker replied.

"It is not love that is an obstacle." said the Siddha. "Desire in love is an obstacle, infatuation is an obstacle. Love is the body of God. The love that you have for yourself and your friends and relations should spread out everywhere. That is the true love that takes you to Ram. Therefore, love everybody."

Do not be angry with the various limbs of your body. If you must be angry, then be angry with anger, not with the body. Listening to what the ignorant say, do not harass the body, which is your companion and friend. Do not deal with it heartlessly or cunningly. Dear seekers! You get the fruit of all actions in the body. The austerities of all the worlds are undergone in the body. All great people have become great in the body. The great seers, sages, kings, heroes, poets, actors, painters, athletes, and warriors, women of great purity, Jesus Christ, Lord Buddha, and all other outstanding people lived in the body. Keep the body pure.

A body that does no work is of no use, so you should make your body disciplined through regular work, *asanas, pranayama,* and meditation. Respect your body as the temple of a deity. Become a priest, offering it the right food and the right relaxation. Let there be only one desire in the body—the desire for love; one wish—to attain the vision of inner light that comes through meditation; one hope—for a body that is moderate and disciplined and radiates inner love. Everything is possible through love. The lover can see God through love, and through love he can easily attain the supremely unattainable. No *sadhana* is as easy as love. This is because you know what love is. It is not something you have to get from outside through *sadhana.* The stream of love is already there inside. You have to spread this love, and in this way it will fill you. The more you give, the more it will grow. He who spreads his love is welcomed with love everywhere.

I have seen many lovers who only hate in the guise of love. There is no place for hatred in love. There should be no feeling of high and low. There are some heartless, angry lovers who say, "We are devotees of Vishnu; we never go to Shiva temples." If you find such anger in love, what kind of love is it? It is really just barbarity. In love there can never be distinctions among castes, people, or religions. Distinctions come from narrowness of vision, not from love. From love comes absorption in non-duality.

Love is within you and gives you ever-new experiences. Think about the contentment of deep sleep. Where does this supersensuous satisfaction come from? When you first meet a friend, you feel satisfaction. Where does that come from? Where does your happiness at the sight of beauty come from? Or the contentment that sometimes arises spontaneously when your mind is filled with joy? Examine all these questions, and you will find that a source of great contentment is hidden within you; it is supremely blissful, and its name is love.

So worship love. Show only scenes of love to the Witness behind your eyes. Let all your acts be full of love. Let your love for cows, trees, flowers, and fruits grow each day, for love is the basis of all.

Love is the mighty nuclear energy that transforms man. So do not let your heart become dry. Do not let every fool you meet convince you that love does not exist within you. Man is unfair to himself because he is ignorant, and when he starts believing he is a sinner and ordinary, he makes other people feel the same. I once went to bathe at the confluence of the three rivers at Allahabad. As I was sitting there, a priest came up and asked me to make a vow. I didn't want to, but he wouldn't listen and kept insisting. He brought flowers and water, saying, "Swamiji, repeat *pāpo'ham*—'I am a sinner.' "

"You're the sinner, not me," I retorted, "even at this holy place you haven't stopped making fools of the pilgrims. I shall say: *puṇyo'ham, puṇyakarmā'ham, saṅkalparahito'ham*—'I am virtuous, I am a doer of good deeds, I am without desire!' " When he heard this, he went away. Through such bad company men are led to believe that they are without joy, that they are unreal, unhappy, poor, and subject to decay, and because they think like this, they cannot let the inner love bloom.

Dear seekers! Learning without love is useless. Yoga without love is meaningless. *Sadhana* without love, whatever *sadhana* it is, cannot take you to the joy of the Self. Fill yourself with love and spread this love among others. Love without desires, craving, or attachment is the key that vanquishes infatuation, enmity, and delusion. You don't have to study a lot of scriptures, because all ideas come from God. Here it is not a question of knowledge but of love.

Don't waste your life getting trapped in arguments about renunciation and acceptance, since they don't have much value. Only knowledge of the Self has value. Yoga, learning, and knowledge, when they are full of egotism, are the enemies of love. You should totally renounce egotism, and this can be done only through love. When selfless love arises in the heart, one experiences deep peace in one's life. Instead of suppressing the mind, fill it with love, then see what marvelous ecstasy there is within yourself.

Instead of torturing your mind through force or breath controls, simply lead it to the Self, pacifying it with love. Let God be the object of all your senses. Tukaram says that the man whose one enjoyment is Narayana sees the world filled with love.

Love is your very nature. It is your *sadhana* and your highest attainment. Love is God; love is the universe. God has appeared as the universe—the universe is no different; it is a manifestation of the divine Shakti. Love is a complete *sadhana* for the realization of God. Without love He cannot be attained.

Love is a great inner experience. Seek it within. You will see the divine Shakti darting with the speed of electricity through your whole body, through all its fluids, blood, prana. As you experience this Shakti, you will know what love is.

The activity inside you always goes on. It never stops. Your nerves, muscles, and blood cells are constantly performing their functions. You should also do your work with love, enthusiasm, and determination, whether you are at home, in an ashram, or elsewhere.

Man should love his Self, which is all-embracing. He should have complete faith in it. Love turns man into an ocean of happiness, an image of peace, a temple of wisdom. Love is man's very Self, his true beauty, and the glory of his human existence. Muktananda says, "First love yourself, then your neighbors, and then the whole world." This is *bhakti;* this is the way to the joy of *jnana;* this is the fulfillment of the joy of yoga. All other *sadhanas* are contained in the *sadhana* of love. Bhagavan Nityananda is that love. He is the supreme bliss that is the reward of all sadhanas. He is adored through the grace of the Guru.

Six

Pleasing the Guru

A Siddha student shouldn't forget that he cannot achieve spiritual perfection through his own efforts. In worldly affairs also, besides making one's own effort, one consults others. One learns from others what one cannot do oneself. In Shaktipat, Kriya Yoga, Siddha Vidya, or Kundalini Maha Yoga, Guru's grace alone is the means of redemption. On this path it is practically impossible to attain perfection without the guidance of the Guru.

Modern ideas on freedom and self-expression are considerable obstacles to Siddha students. If the student of the Siddha Path abuses the word "freedom" and is lazy or negligent about obeying the Guru, if he looks for faults in him or has little faith, he finds that the Shakti is destroyed after a while. When a king comes to stay in a house, he comes with all his pomp and magnificence. He makes the house rich and grand. He diffuses pleasure, beauty, and greatness to every corner of the house. But when he leaves, he takes all his glory with him, and the house is left empty of radiance and beauty. Will the all-knowing Shakti, which is actively functioning in the seeker, which has been received from the Guru, and which works under the Guru's direction, be pleased to stay with the Siddha student who harbors suspicions about the Guru, seeing faults in him and arguing with himself about the Guru? On the path of the Siddhas, in Kundalini Mahayoga: *gurukripā hi kevalam gurorājnā hi kevalam*—"Only the grace of the

Guru, only the command of the Guru matters." What Muktananda says is true: "The grace of the Guru is the most important thing in all knowledge, liberation, and inquiry into the true nature of the Self." Jnaneshwar Maharaj says that your efforts, your repetition of mantras, your austerities, your yoga, and your *sadhana* bear fruit only when the time comes for you to receive the Guru's grace. *Sadhakas* should remember that the Guru will stand by them with just as much glory, excellence, perfection, and power as they attribute to him. The contraction and expansion of your Shakti, the progress or retardation of your *sadhana*, and the time of its culmination all depend on the intensity of your feeling. In truth, the stronger and more intense your feeling for the Guru as God-incarnate, the sooner you will attain everything. It won't take you any time. I shall describe a small incident that may increase the *sadhaka's* faith and devotion and help him to reach his goal.

In Mahableshwar a student of the Indian Institute of Technology came to see me. Within four days of his arrival he received grace, began to do *sadhana*, and started to meditate very well. Then the time came for him to return to Bombay. Because of the rains his bus was delayed, and when midnight came he was still on the road. Meanwhile, in Bombay, his mother had been waiting anxiously for him, wondering why the bus hadn't arrived. At 10:00 she stopped thinking of her dear son and, instead, started her prayers to her Gurudev. As she prayed, she became absorbed in *gurubhava*. Then her Guru appeared before her and said, "Mother, don't worry. Your son will get home at 12:25." When she heard this, she stopped worrying completely. Because of her faith, the Guru revealed himself to her and she stopped watching for her son. She again sank deep into meditation. After a time she heard someone knocking on the door, calling, "Mother, Mother." She got up and opened the door. Her son was standing there. She looked at the clock; it was exactly 12:25. She was overcome with wonder. Later she came to Mahableshwar herself, and when I heard the whole episode from her, I was inspired to write this chapter on "Pleasing the Guru."

Saint Tukaram, the ever-to-be-remembered inhabitant of Siddhaloka, wrote a song on pleasing the Guru, which I am quoting here for the help of Siddha students:

gurucharaṇī ṭhevitā bhāva āpe āpa bheṭe deva
mhaṇunī gurusī bhajāve svadyānāsī āṇāve
deva gurupāsī āhe vāraṁvāra sāṅgūṁ kāye
tukā mhaṇe gurubhajanī deva bheṭe janīṁ vanīṁ

It means that when you put all your heart and all your faith in the Guru's feet you meet God without any effort—it happens of its own accord. So praise the Guru, bring him into your meditation. God lives with the Guru. How often must I say it? Tukaram says that when you praise the Guru you can meet God in the world as well as in a forest. So, dear Siddha students, remember that you must have complete and ideal faith in and absolute devotion to the feet of the Guru.

Bhava, feeling, is something very wonderful. Once you have established a *bhava*, if you turn it around, the same *bhava* can become its opposite. Your *bhava* should be such that it makes you grow. This is called abiding faith. For the Siddha student who has experienced even once the divine power and influence of the dynamic Chiti Shakti, a deep and abiding faith arises in the Chiti Shakti now manifest within him, in his Guru, in his own Self, and in the universe as the field of the play of divine Consciousness. It then becomes very difficult for his mind, thoughts, and intellect to abandon the inner Chiti Shakti, his devout feeling for his Guru and his inner Self, and wander here and there for no reason. He finds no happiness or sorrow in the condition and states of the world, which momentarily arise and subside. Truly, you must have firm, total devotion and confidence in the Guru.

To describe the kind of faith one should have in the omnipotence of God and in the power of the inner Consciousness, I shall tell the story of Prahlada, a sage born in a family of demons. The story of this king of devotees is well known to Indians. Hiranyakashipu, the father of Prahlada and king of the demons, tried many times to get his son to give up his devotion to Vishnu and to follow the ways and customs of the demons. Prahlada neither gave up his devotion nor did he learn the ways of the demons. What does the man who has had a full realization of the divine power in his heart have to fear? When Chiti is playing within him, what can he lack? Eventually, Hiranyakashipu got tired of trying to persuade Prahlada. He flew into a rage and cried, "The earth splits asunder and the winds stop blowing at my solemn words, but this boy disregards them! The silly little child won't eat, dance, hunt, and enjoy himself as we've always done in our family, but has got into bad company and instead runs off to meditate on God. He has fallen from our religion and he is a disgrace to our family traditions. It would be better to have no son than to have a degenerate one like this." In his rage, Hiranyakashipu roared like a lion. He summoned a multitude of demons, who came running to him with their weapons. The king of the demons said, "This is my command—cut Prahlada to pieces!" The demons at once bared their weapons and set out to find Prahlada, each one ready to slice off his head. When the devout Prahlada saw the demons bearing down upon him with weapons raised to strike, he felt no fear at all and said:

> *viṣṇuḥ śastreṣu yuṣmāsu mayi chāsau vyavasthitaḥ*
> *daiteyāstena satyena mākramantvāyudhāni cha*
>
> (*Vishnu Purana* 1:17/33)

O demons, my Lord Vishnu is in these weapons, he is in you, and he is in me. The all-pervading Vishnu is in my father, too. He is everywhere.

"*Vasudevah sarvamiti*—Vasudeva is indeed all. This is the supreme truth. Truth is eternal. It is perfect and supremely fearless. By the power of this great truth, by my unmoving faith and devotion I see all-pervasive Vishnu in you and in the edges of your swords. Your weapons won't have any power over me because of this faith." Having said these words, he stood there quite calmly. Prahlada felt no pain at all when the weapons of the demons struck him. As each weapon touched him it wrapped itself around him like a garland of flowers. His inner state did not change. His meditation was not disturbed at all. He did not blame anyone for what was happening and was not agitated by anything, as he had given himself completely to Vishnu. Prahlada's joy, his suffering, his anxiety, his grief—all were Vishnu. Indeed, one who claims to have surrendered everything to God and yet weeps is an imposter among devotees and is just making a business of devotion. He is far from the Truth, and his devotion is simply play-acting.

If a man has the devotion to his Guru that Prahlada had for Vishnu, it is not at all amazing that God should reveal Himself to him from within. This is why Tukaram Maharaj says that God is easily found when one has unwavering faith in the feet of the Guru, since God dwells with the Guru. Muktananda says: By the love of the Guru, by the grace of the Guru, *sadhana* came searching for me; I didn't look for it. *Bandhas, mudras,* and *kriyas* came to me; I didn't invite them. The people who live in the Ashram and the people with the arts and skills required to run it came looking for me; I didn't run after them. I only ran after my Guru. I was always ready to obey the command of my Guru. I followed the path he showed me, never wondering when I would reach perfection, never asking where the road was leading. Whatever path he put me on, I followed, regarding it as his command. Since I followed in that way, I reached where I should have reached. I didn't look to one side or the other, nor did I bother about small things. I just kept going straight ahead. I found what I had to find. I became what I was to become, and in the becoming there was nothing lacking.

Dear Siddha students, first I did it, now I am telling you. A sage once said:

śrīgurucharaṇāmbhojaṁ satyameva vijānatām
jagata satyamasatyaṁ vā netareti matirmama

Know the lotus feet of the Guru as the Truth. Then you don't have to think about whether the world is real or unreal.

O seekers! Leave these questions to the scholars. On the theme of the Guru's feet, Sri Jnaneshwar Maharaj says to the Siddha student in search of happiness:

O Sadguru! When a *sadhaka* worships your two feet—*tat* and *twam*—with *asi,* "Thou art That," there is nothing left for him to attain.

Dear Siddha students! Honor the Guru with all your heart. Worship him with all your heart. Love him with all your heart. All the supernatural powers will come to you, will stand in attendance ready to serve you. You won't have to display little miracles like a magician.

The *Nigama* scriptures say:

gurusantoṣamātreṇa siddhirbhavati śāsvatī
anyathā naiva siddhiḥ syādabhichārāya kalpate

Everlasting divine power is obtained only when the Guru is pleased. Otherwise there will be no true power but only a short-lived *siddhi*.

No matter how much you repeat mantras, how much *tapasya* you practice, how long you meditate, how much you give in charity, how many sacrifices you offer, or how many times you bathe in the Ganges, you cannot attain anything without the Guru's favor.

The weakness, carelessness, and lack of enthusiasm that one sees among today's Siddha students comes from the fact that they have not pleased the Guru. The grace of the Guru inspires the intellect, destroys sorrows, and gives one an avid interest in *sadhana*. By the Guru's grace alone, one finds pleasure in repeating God's name, so that yogic *kriyas* start happening of their own accord. By the Guru's grace you find *samadhi* in your daily life and see God in the world. So remember to please the Guru. If one tiny spark from the fire of the Guru's grace falls on the disciple, a divine mood will arise within. The wish-fulfilling tree, the wish-fulfilling gem, and the wish-fulfilling cow are nothing compared with the Sadguru filled with universal Consciousness. Sundardas sings of the glory of such a Guru:

> *gurudeva sarvopari adhika birājamāna*
> *gurudeva sabahi teṁ adhika gariṣṭha hai*
> *gurudeva dattātreya nārada śukādi muni*
> *gurudeva gyānadhana pragaṭa vasiṣṭha hai*
> *gurudeva parama ānandamaya dekhiyata*
> *gurudeva vara vari-yāna hū variṣṭha hai*
> *suṅdara kahata kachhu mahimā kahī na jāye*
> *aise gurudeva dādū mere sira iṣṭa haiṁ*

Gurudeva is above everyone; he is most brilliant; he is greater than all.

Gurudeva is Dattatreya, Narada, Shuka, and other sages; he is the treasure of wisdom; the sage Vasishtha manifest.

Gurudeva appears full of supreme bliss; he is great, greater, greatest.

Sundar is unable to tell his glory.

Such a Gurudev is Dadu, my most adorable deity.

Whoever has attained spiritual perfection has done so through his Guru. The Guru grants a life full of grace, complete freedom, and liberation of the Self. The Guru's favor is absolutely necessary for lasting attainment. Without a Guru man is unhappy; with a Guru he is full of joy. So surrender yourself completely to the Guru, and embrace true *gurubhava*. To have meditated a little, to have had a few *kriyas* and seen a few lights, is not *gurubhava*. Indeed, *gurubhava* is far from this. The more your *bhava* is developed, the higher the level of spiritual evolution you will reach.

> *deve tīrthe dvije mantre daivajne bheṣaje gurau*
> *yādraśī bhāvanā yasya siddhirbhavati tādraśī*

The benefit obtained from gods, holy places, brahmins, mantras, divine beings, herbs, and the Guru is directly proportional to the quality of one's feeling for them.

Decide for yourself what your behavior should be toward the Guru, who saves those sinking into the ocean of worldliness and makes them like himself, who enters his disciple and fills him with Chiti to remove all his doubts, who illumines his heart with the light of God; who awakens the divine radiance of his disciple's Self and gives him the delight of the Self just like his own.

Truly, the Guru has the power to make the disciple's world full of divine Consciousness. If a man does not see this play of Consciousness, then no matter what he does, he cannot find supreme peace. He may practice yoga, sacrifices, and mantras, but he will not find the peace that should be their fruit. He may follow the code of restraints and observances and wander from one holy place to another, but he will attain nothing; he will only reduce his life. He may eat only roots and fruits all his life, acquire supernatural powers, practice severe asceticism, worship the different gods and goddesses, perform meritorious acts, but still he will not find peace and happiness if he has not seen *chitshakti vilas*, the play of divine Consciousness, through the grace of Guru. Sri Abhinavaguptacharya says:

> *svatantraḥ svachchhātmā sphurati satataṁ chetasi śivaḥ*
> *parāśaktischeyaṁ karaṇasaraṇiprāntamuditā*
> *tadā bhogaikātmā sphurati cha samastaṁ jagadidam*
> *na jāne kutrāyaṁ dhvaniranupatet saṁsritiriti*

Shiva, the independent and pure Self that always vibrates in the mind, is the Parashakti that rises as joy in various sense experiences. Then the experience of this outer world appears as its Self. I do not know from where this word *"samsara"* has come.

This supremely pure, conscious Self—whom people call Parameshvara, Krishna, Rama, Shiva, Jagadamba, Mother of the world, Brahman, Chaitanya or pure Consciousness, *nirguna, saguna*, Allah, God, Satnam, or Alakh; whom Muktananda calls Nityananda; whom the *Pratyabhijnahridayam* calls Chitshakti; and whom the Siddhas call Kundalini—this supremely free Parashiva vibrates constantly in every mind. This same Being, as Parashakti, wells up with the same joy that the various senses experience through their own activities. The same universal Self, whose nature is Being, Consciousness, and Bliss, is manifesting itself as the whole universe. It is this Chiti Shakti who, living in the heart of every Siddha student, experiences and enjoys the world, which is permeated with Chiti. I don't understand how it came to be supposed that the universe was one thing, the living individual being a second, and *maya* a third; there is nothing besides Chiti that has the capacity to manifest as the world. What can mar that Chiti who is absolutely independent and pure in Her radiance? Who could stay beside a blazing fire? The whole universe is the play of Chiti.

To help you understand the *chitivilas*, the play of Chiti, I quote some poetry that describes how the *gopis*, the milkmaids of Vraja, saw the *chitivilas* as a *krishnavilas*, a play of Krishna, a sport full of His glory:

jita dekhau tita syāmamaī hai
syāma kuṅja bana jamunā syāmā syāma gagana ghanaghatā chhaī hai
saba raṅgana meṁ syāma bharo hai loka kahata yah bāta naī hai
maiṁ baurī kī logana hī kī syāma putariyā badala gaī hai

> Wherever the eyes may fall, Krishna is all they see;
> The bowers, the forests and the river Yamuna,
> The sky and the dark clouds,
> All the different colors are full of Krishna.
> People exclaim, 'This is a new idea!'
> Whether I am mad or they are blind I cannot decide.

kahi na jāya mukhasau kachū syāma-premakī bāta
nabha jala thala chara achara saba syāmahi syāma dikhāta
brahma nahīm māyā nahīm nahīm jīva nahīm kāla
apanīhū sudhi nā rahī rahyo eka nandalāla
ko kāso kehi bidhi kahā kahai hridaikī bāta
hari herata hiya hari gayo hari sarvatra lakhāta

The love of Krishna is beyond words;
I see Him, only Him in the sky and water and lands,
In the animate and the inanimate.
Neither Brahman nor *maya* exist, neither the individual soul
            nor time;
Nor am I conscious of myself; all that is, is Krishna, the son
            of Nanda.
How can I ever express the longing of my heart?
Who can? In what way?
I thought I could possess Hari, but He possessed my heart.
I see Him everywhere, in all directions.

The whole universe is the playground of Chiti, it is the manifestation of God, it is the splendor of the true Self of the Siddha student.
It is completely pervaded by Sri Gurudev. This is why there has been
so much emphasis in this chapter on how one should understand the
Guru. You should be really attentive to this. The *chitshakti vilas*,
the play of the power of Consciousness, is the universal form of the
Guru. This same power becomes the Sadguru and bestows knowledge,
and it becomes the disciple and receives knowledge. This power assumes innumerable bodies. The same Sadguru enters all beings as
prana. He becomes Brahma, Vishnu, and Rudra. He becomes celestial
beings like Varuna, Indra, the sun and the moon, the seven planets,
Rahu and Ketu, the Pole Star, and the constellation of the Great Bear.
He becomes all these things, and yet retains his own unity. The Guru
is the speaker and what is spoken, the hearer and what is heard, the
knower and what is known. He is the *Vedas* and the knower of the
Vedas. He is the Sankhya philosophy, he is yoga and the actions of
yoga, he is Yogesh, the lord of yoga. He becomes all things and still
is one. Sri Guru is the doer, the instruments of actions, and the deed.
He is the experiencer, the objects of experience, and the experience.
He is the elixir of immortality, medicines, disease, and death. The

same One pervades all beings—ignorant and enlightened, undiscerning and wise, man and god. Numbers and mathematics are the vibration of the Self. All *ragas* and *raginis*, all rhythms and sounds are made from Him. He is the dancer and the tuneful singer. He is the dance and the song. The same perfect Sadguru is the teacher of pure knowledge and the founder of Maha Yoga and the Siddha Science. The scriptures say of him: *manuṣyadehamāsthāya chhannāsate parameśvarāḥ*—"Almighty God conceals Himself in a human form as the Guru."

Dear Siddha students desirous of liberation! This whole universe is the glory of the Guru. It is the expansion of your own Self. This is the teaching of the Siddhas, the teaching of Sri Guru, the view of Vedanta, and the experience of saints and mystics. If you see any duality in this play of divine Consciousness, you will remain far from happiness, you will find no contentment or joy. You will never be liberated from the pain of birth and death. Srimat Shankaracharya says:

svalpamapyantaraṁ krutvā jīvātmaparamātmanoḥ
yaḥ saṁtiṣṭhati mūḍhātma bhayaṁ tasyābhibhāṣitam

The foolish being who lives making even the slightest distinction between the supreme Self and his own Self will always be subject to fear.

Whether it is through the reading of incorrect scriptures, through bad company, or through the delusion of the differentiating mentality, the man who sees and accepts the slightest difference between God, the individual soul, and himself will always be afraid; he will never find peace. It is said in the *Upanishads: dvitīyādvai bhayaṁ bhavati* —"He who sees another will be in fear." He who regards the all-pervasive universe as different from himself, from his Guru, from God, and from Chiti Shakti Kundalini will always be afraid; he will never find peace.

yathā nyagrodhabījasthaḥ śaktirūpo mahādrumaḥ
tathā hridayabījasthaṁ viśvametachcharācharam

Just as the tiniest seed grows into a strong, huge, sprawling banyan tree, so does the power of the soul, embedded in the heart in seed form, expand into the animate and inanimate universe.

So, dear Siddha students, always remember: *gurusantoṣamātreṇa siddhirbhavati śāsvatī*—"The root of all attainments and of everlasting peace is the pleasing of the Guru."

When is the Guru pleased? Don't think that you can satisfy him by standing in front of him and praising him to his face saying, "What a great Guru!" If you meditate a little bit once a week but spend the next twenty days going to the cinema and then exclaim, "What a great Guru!" don't think you are pleasing him. If you meditate a little once in a fortnight, but spend a month wandering the streets like a vagabond and then exclaim, "What a great Guru!" don't think you are pleasing him. If you meditate once in a month, but spoil and rot your stomach by eating *bhelpuris* for three months and then exclaim, "What a great Guru!" don't think you are pleasing him. The Guru is not going to be very pleased with all that. The Guru is pleased when his disciple attains perfection. Just as an artist praises his student and gives his blessing when he has mastered his art, just as an athlete praises his student when he too becomes an athlete or a scholar blesses his student for his scholarship, so the Guru is pleased when his disciple, on whom he has bestowed his Shakti, attains perfection. You can never please the Guru by giving him clothes and money, by feeding and praising him to his face.

The Guru is pleased when the disciple merges with him and becomes the Guru. Thus Muktananda says:

> I go to the Guru for refuge.
> I go to the yoga of meditation for refuge.
> I attain love and devotion for the Guru.
> I take as mine the motto "See the divine in others."
> I remember the Guru always.
> The Guru is my mind; the Guru is my journey and my goal;
> The Guru is my delight; the Guru is my Self.
> This, I say, is the truth, the truth.

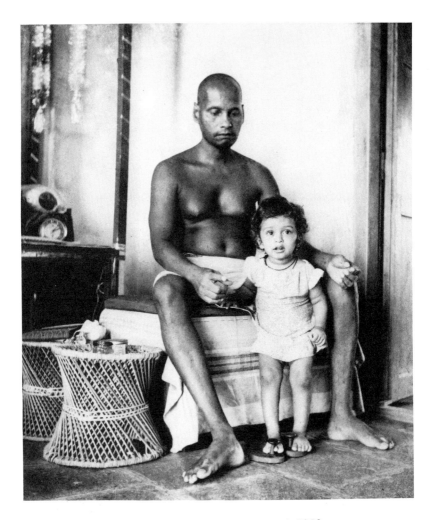

Swami Muktananda in Ganeshpuri, 1958

In the *Pratyabhijnahridayam* there is an aphorism: *madhyavikāsāt chidānandalābhaḥ,* which means that when, through the grace of a Siddha, the Kundalini rises in the *sushumna* of the Siddha student, he obtains the knowledge of the Goddess Chiti. Through meditation his mind remains in a state of equanimity and the perfect knowledge of Chiti arises from within. Subsequently, the state that he experiences in meditation persists in his everyday life. Such a yogi becomes totally serene in his meditation, and in his worldly life becomes totally free from anxiety. This yogic state gradually becomes firm, and soon he lives in a state of imperturbability. As a fruit of the *sadhana* done by Guru's grace, Chiti Shakti of Her own accord assumes this state within the yogi. It is called *sahajavastha,* or the state of pure spontaneity. A man who is in *sahajavastha* is known as a *mahayogi,* or a supreme devotee of Shiva, even if he lives in the world. He can see the blossoming of Chiti in all the deeds and actions of his daily life, in his worship, in chanting and meditation, in his house, his children, his servants, and in everything he eats and drinks.

This man sees the everlasting play of Chiti within and without—*sabāhyābhyāntaraḥ ayaṁ nityoditasamāveśātmā.* As he sees this, complete equanimity comes to his mind. This is *sahajavastha,* the state of pure spontaneity. In this unchangeable state, endowed with the force of the great mantra, he loses the feeling that his body, his *prana,* and his senses and their objects are different from his own Self. To him they are all pervaded by Chiti. He is inspired with the feeling that however he may conceive of them, it is the great and glorious Chiti Shakti who is the basis of them all.

Without the vibrations of Chiti, no object could be perceived. By Her existence She reveals all objects. In this way, it is the same Chiti Shakti that sports in all states, enters into all matter, and absorbs everything into Her own being. The One whose light streams through brilliant objects is the same One who becomes space, time, and form. Chiti Shakti illuminates every material object in the phenomenal universe. All things within and without are created, sustained, and pass away in this Shakti. By seeing his mind and his external organs as Her rays, the Siddha student or Siddha yogi experiences Godhood, and on discovering this, his mind attains peace and equanimity. This is the state of *sahajavastha,* of pure spontaneity, of natural *samadhi.* The yogi in this state understands God as the one who appears in an infinity of forms, who is the whole and indivisible support of the phenomenal universe, and who also pervades all physical objects and all living creatures. This man experiences the continual influence of God in all that he does. Just as the shape of a fruit, its juice, its smell, and all its various characteristics exist as a simple unity, so the yogi discovers that external objects, the knowledge of these objects, and the one who knows them are all one with the all-pervading God, the fundamental basis of all things. Thus, the yogi discovers this in everyone. When this is discovered, the idea *alpo'ham*—"I am insignificant," is destroyed in the Siddha student, and in its place comes the knowledge *purno'ham*—"I am perfect." This is spontaneous *samadhi.*

In fact, all phenomenal appearance is nothing but Chiti. For the Siddha student there is nothing in the universe other than Chiti. Sri Shankaracharya says:

> *rajjvajnānāt kshaṇenaiva yadvadrajjurhi sarpiṇī*
> *bhāti tadvachchitiḥ sākshādviśvākāreṇa kevalā*
>
> (*Aparokshanubhuti,* 44)

> Just as, through ignorance of the real nature of a rope, it may for a moment appear to be a snake, so does pure Consciousness appear in the form of the phenomenal universe without undergoing any change.

A man in his confusion may mistake a rope for a snake. He may react by fainting or his heart may miss a beat and he may start shouting, "Run! Run!" But then a wise man comes, who knows what a rope is. He says, "O ignorant one! Why are you shouting and getting upset? It's not a snake; it's only a rope." After hearing this, the same man will see a rope instead of the snake he saw earlier. Just as a snake had appeared in the rope, in the same way the universe appears in Chiti.

> *brahmaiva sarvanāmāni rūpāni vividhāni cha*
> *karmānyapi samagrāni bibhartīti śrutirjagau*
>
> (*Aparokshanubhuti,* 50)

The *Vedas* have clearly declared that Brahman alone is the substratum of all varieties of names, forms, and actions.

Truly all the various things in the universe, all the names that correspond to them, and their functions—the seeing of eyes, the grasping of hands, the speaking of tongues, and so on—are all assumed by God. Furthermore:

> *sarvo'pi vyavahārastu brahmanā kriyate janaih*
> *ajnānānna vijānanti mradeva hi ghatādikam*

The actions of all people are performed by Brahman. It is only because of ignorance that one does not perceive clay in pots and other objects.

Everything done by man is effected by the existence of God. Nothing could happen without God. The radio speaks, but behind it is the power of electricity. Without this power it is inert. Similarly, everything that is done by the senses and the organs is done because there is the conscious Self, or Chiti, behind them. Ignorant people who have not received the wisdom of the Guru think that the eyes see, the tongue speaks, and the legs move, that the senses are quite independent in what they do. When there is no electricity, the radio does not play; in the same way, when the conscious Self leaves the body, the eyes do not see and the tongue does not speak. This is why Shankaracharya says that everything happens by virtue of the existence of the conscious Self. Chiti speaks as the tongue's tongue, sees as the eye's eye, hears as the ear's ear, and thinks as the mind's mind. To live with the understanding that one universal Consciousness plays in the functions of every part of man's being, in every movement of the inner and outer universe, to be free from the distinction of unity and multiplicity, and to remain serene is *sahajavastha.*

Students of meditation know through experience that once their meditation becomes pure it becomes free from thought. For example, when your meditation is fixed on the Blue Pearl, the mind becomes permeated by it and, in fact, becomes it. You temporarily lose consciousness of yourself; you become oblivious of the inner and outer worlds: objects are not seen when there is no one to see them, and sounds are not heard when there is no one to hear them. In that state there is neither happiness nor sorrow nor ignorance, neither perceiver nor perceived. Only the pure Paramatma, the supreme Self, remains, pulsating in His own being. It is an unwavering, thought-free, tranquil condition. It is the goal of your meditation. A man stays in this state for a short time, and then, when he begins to come out of meditation, he goes from *turiyatita* into the *turiya* state. Afterward, in *turiya,* no matter what happens, he will retain the realization of the transcendental state of *turiyatita.* Then, passing from *turiya* into *sushupti,* or deep sleep, he takes with him the experience of the *turiya* state. In deep sleep he still sees nothing different from himself. Leaving deep sleep and going into the dream state, he becomes his own dream world and all the objects of that state—chariots, horses, elephants, etc. He discovers that the Witness of the deep sleep state is the same as that of dreams. And then, passing from the dreaming to the waking state, he realizes that the same transcendental Being also underlies that. Thus from *turiyatita* to *turiya, turiya* to deep sleep, deep sleep to dreaming, dreaming to waking—and vice versa—only one Witness remains. The four states may differ from each other in various ways, but the Witness of them is the same. To become peaceful by understanding that there is one Witness of all the four states is, according to Muktananda, *sahajavastha.*

There is a state of non-recognition of Chiti Shakti. In that condition all the things of the universe appear to man as different. He identifies their forms, names, qualities, functions, and so on and thinks that they are many. With the insight received from the Guru, he gains the knowledge of the Chiti Shakti:

sa chaiko dvirūpastrimayaśchaturātmā saptapanchakasvabhāvaḥ

(Pratyabhijnahridayam, 7)

This aphorism means that the one Paramashiva becomes the universe by becoming two, three, four, and thirty-six elements. He is the attributeless and formless Satchidananada. When the same Satchidananda expands and contracts, He is said to become two. When He assumes the limitations of individualization, differentiation, and action (*anava, mayiya,* and *karma*), He is termed "threefold." When He assumes the four divisions of *shunya* (void), *prana, puryashtaka* (the "city of eight"—the five senses and the mind, intellect, and ego), and the physical body, He is known as the "fourfold soul." He becomes the thirty-six elements of manifestation, right from Parashiva to the physical earth. But He is still one. There is nothing other than He. The *Pratyabhijnahridayam* says that the whole world is the play of Chiti:

chidātmā śivabhattaraka eva eka ātmā na tu anyaḥ kaśchita

There is only one Self, the conscious Self, Lord Shiva; nothing else exists.

As this is understood, the fluctuations of the mind cease, and this is *sahajavastha.* The *Vijnanabhairava* says:

grāhyagrāhakasaṁvittiḥ sāmānya sarvadehināma
yogināṁ tu viśeṣo'yaṁ sambandhe sāvadhānatā

Knowledge of the perceiver and the perceived is common to all beings, but with yogis it is different. They are aware of them as one.

Parashakti, the Goddess Chiti, becomes both the phenomenal universe that can be seen and the *jivatma,* the individual being who feels himself to be different from the universe. The perceived is termed *grahya,* and means the universe and all its objects. The perceiver is termed *grahaka,* and means the *jivatma,* the conscious individual soul, the knower of these objects. Ignorant or ordinary people split the perceiver and the perceived into countless different divisions. But a yogi, a worshiper of

Maha Yoga blessed by the Guru's grace, having realized Chitshakti, becomes aware that both the perceiver and the perceived have sprung from Her; thus, he sees them equally. The peace and equanimity that come to a yogi with the realization of this sameness is the state of *sahaja*.

Wise people see the world as the play of universal Consciousness. They call it the vibrating of Chiti. They know that Chiti appears as the ordinary world. The world born from Chiti may assume different forms, but it is one Chiti. All giving and taking, all activities, are the expansion of Chiti. She assumes infinite forms within Herself and then expands in all those form. To understand this, and to be peaceful, is Muktananda's state of *sahaja*. *Iti Shivam.*

Benediction

My dear, my own Siddha students!

May your meditation, by the power of the Siddha Science and by the grace of a Siddha, become totally established in the repose of the Siddhas, even while you remain engaged in your daily activities. This is my blessing.

Beloved Siddha students! Having been worthy of receiving the grace of a Siddha, you now belong to the Siddha lineage. Your world is Siddhaloka. Your state is the same as that attained by the Siddhas. The most divine power of grace of countless great beings living in Siddhaloka stands behind you to protect you. May you be fully protected by this power of grace. This is my blessing.

Siddha students! Only a few sparks of fire can burn an entire forest to ashes. Similarly, even the tiny ray of the Siddhas' Chiti Shakti that has entered you burns away your impurities. May it grant you perfect Siddhahood. This is my blessing.

You are all rays of Siddha beings. You are all taking part in the play of Chiti Shakti. She is active within you. May you become saturated with Consciousness in the world you live in, which is also the embodiment of Consciousness and, merging in Chiti, become Chiti. May your minds attain complete repose in the Goddess Chiti's realm, which is nothing but stillness. This is my blessing.

My supreme Guru, Sri Nityananda, is also my supreme deity. He is the image of Chiti and abides in Siddhaloka. With just a small portion of his grace, I erased my individuality and became the expansion and pulsation of Kundalini, who is nothing but Chiti. He selflessly took away all my pain and suffering, and in their place gave me his own being. To protect the Shakti that he had given me, he himself became Shakti and took seat within me as my own Self, becoming the Master of my heart. Because of him, I am. I am his; he created me. May Lord Sri Guru Nityananda, whom I worship constantly, the inner Self of all, the activator of Shakti and the chakras, enter into all my Siddha students, residing within them as their inner Self. May he fill their lives with bliss. This is my blessing.

Revered Sri Nityananda's own,

Beloved Sri Siddha student's own,

Swami Muktananda

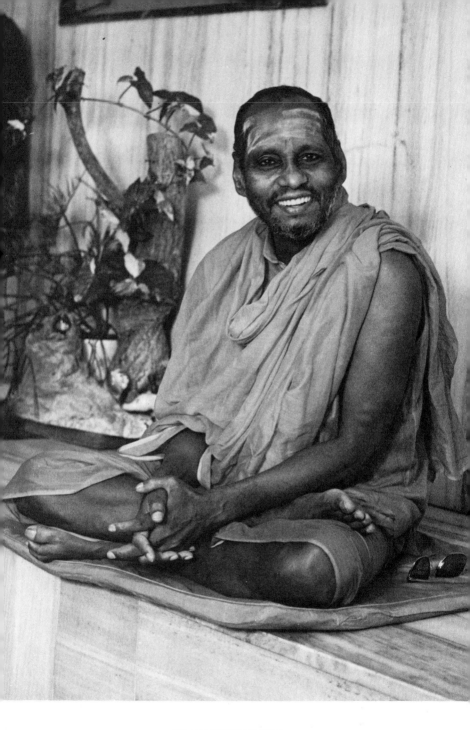

Swami Muktananda

---

abhanga: a devotional song composed in the Marathi language.

abhaya mudra: a symbolic gesture formed by raising one hand with the palm outward, meaning "Do not fear." Many deities, saints, and idols are pictured with this gesture. *see also: mudra.*

Ajamila: a *brahmin* who fell from his life of pure conduct when he was aroused by passion for a woman. But by invoking the name of God at the time of his death, he was redeemed, and was taken to heaven by messengers of Vishnu.

ajna chakra: the spiritual center located between the eyebrows. The awakened Kundalini passes through this *chakra* only by the command (*ajna*) of the Guru, and for this reason it is also known as the *guru chakra.* When Shaktipat is given, the Guru often touches the seeker at this spot. *see also: chakra.*

akasha: ether, the subtlest of the five elements, which gives rise to the other four elements and which has the attribute of all-pervasiveness. *see also*: five elements.

Akrura: Krishna's uncle.

Allahabad (*or*: Prayag):   a holy center at the confluence of three sacred rivers of India—the Ganges, Jamuna, and Saraswati. The confluence, called *triveni*, is an important sacred spot and a place of pilgrimage. It is one of the sites of the *kumbha mela*, a spiritual festival where hundreds of thousands of devotees from all over India gather.

Aparokshanubhuti: a work on Vedanta by Shankaracharya explaining God-realization as an immediate and direct perception of one's own Self by means of inquiry.

arati: the waving of lights, incense, camphor, and other things before a saint or idol as an act of worship.

Arjuna: the third of the five Pandava brothers and one of the heroes of the *Mahabharata* epic. It was to Arjuna that Krishna imparted the knowledge of the *Bhagavad Gita.*

asana: various bodily postures, practiced to strengthen the body, purify the nerves, and develop one-pointedness of mind—the yoga scriptures describe eighty-four major *asanas*; a seat or mat on which one sits for meditation. *see also*: eight limbs of yoga.

ashram: a spiritual institution or community where spiritual discipline is practiced; the abode of a saint or holy man.

ashramas: the four stages of traditional Hindu life. They are: *brahmacharyashrama*, the stage of a student engaged in scriptural study and the practice of celibacy; *grahasthashrama,* the stage of a householder engaged in leading a family life; *vanaprasthashrama,* the stage of retirement when one engages in scriptural study and other spiritual practices; and *sannyasashrama,* the stage of complete renunciation in which one is freed from all worldly obligations and responsibilities in order to devote one's life to the pursuit of Self-realization.

ashtagandha: a tree whose seeds are dried and crushed into an orange powder, which is then mixed with sandal paste and applied to the forehead during worship.

avadhuta: a saint who has transcended body-consciousness and whose behavior is not bound by ordinary social conventions.

Ayurveda (*lit.* knowledge of life):   ancient Indian science of medicine which teaches that good health depends on maintaining the even balance of the three bodily humours: wind, bile and phlegm.

Ayodhya: birthplace of Rama in North India, which today is a center of pilgrimage.

Baba: a term of affection for a saint or holy man, meaning "father."

Badrinath: one of the major centers of pilgrimage, sacred to Vishnu, located in the heart of the Himalayas.

Baglamukhi (*lit.* crane-headed):   an aspect of the universal Mother (Shakti) who is depicted with the head of a crane.

bhakta: a devotee, a lover of God; a follower of Bhakti Yoga—the path of love and devotion.

bhakti (Bhakti Yoga):   the path of devotion leading to union with God; the state of intense devotional love for God or Guru.

bandha (*lit.* bondage): a class of exercises in Hatha Yoga, which when practiced along with *pranayama* (breathing exercises) aids in uniting the *prana* and *apana* (the ingoing and outgoing breath). They also help to seal the *prana* in the body during the practice of *mudras*. There are three major *bandhas: jalandhara, mula,* and *uddiyana.*

Bhagavan: the Lord; a term of address for God or saints denoting the glorious, divine, venerable, and holy.

bhajiya: Indian snack made from gram flour, spices, and vegetables fried in oil.

bhava: emotion; feeling of absorption or identification; spiritual attitude.

Bhavani: one of the names of the universal Mother, meaning "the giver of existence."

Bhishma: the partiarch of the Kaurava and Pandava families, whose story is told in the *Mahabharata* epic.

bhujangini mudra: a Hatha Yoga exercise, called the serpent *mudra,* in which one draws in air through the esophagus. Its practice destroys stomach disease. *see also: mudra.*

Brahma: the Absolute Reality manifested as the active creator of the universe, who is personified as one of the three gods of the Hindu trinity. The other two are: Vishnu, who represents the principle of sustenance, and Shiva, who represents the principle of destruction.

Brahman (*or*: Brahma): the Absolute Reality or all-pervasive supreme principle of the universe. The nature of Brahman is described in the *Upanishads* and in Vedantic philosophy as: *sat* (Existence absolute), *chit* (Consciousness absolute), and *ananda* (Bliss absolute). *see also: satchidananda.*

brahmabhava: identification with the all-pervasive Reality.

brahmacharya: *see: ashramas.*

brahmamuhurta: the period of time between 3:00 A.M. and 6:00 A.M., supposed to be the best time for meditation and worship.

brahmarandhra (*lit.* the hole of Brahman): a subtle center located in the crown of the head.

brahmin: the first caste of Hindu society, the members of which are by tradition priests and scholars. *see also*: caste.

caste: ancient Indian society was organized into four *varnas* (divisions or castes): *brahmins* (scholars, priests, preceptors); *kshatriyas* (rulers and warriors); *vaishyas* (business and agricultural classes);

and *shudras* (menial laborers).

chakra (*lit.* wheel): a center of energy located in the subtle body where the *nadis* (channels) converge, giving the appearance of a lotus. There are six main *chakras* located in the *sushumna* (the subtle central channel). The *chakras* are centers of consciousness within man which control the functions of all the nerves of the body. The Kundalini lies dormant, coiled at the base of the *sushumna* in the *muladhara chakra.* When awakened, either by yogic practices or by Guru's grace, Kundalini begins to ascend through the *sushumna* piercing all the *chakras* until She enters the *sahasrara,* the topmost spiritual center. The six main *chakras* are: 1. *muladhara*: a four-petaled lotus located at the base of the spinal column, where Kundalini lies coiled up.

2. *svadhishthana*: a six-petaled lotus located at the root of the reproductive organs.

3. *manipura*: a ten-petaled lotus located in the naval region.

4. *anahata*: a twelve-petaled lotus located in the region of the heart.

5. *vishuddha*: a sixteen-petaled lotus located at the base of the throat.

6. *ajna*: a two-petaled lotus located between the two eyebrows, a seat of the Guru.

Chanur: a wrestler in Kamsa's court who was ordered to kill Krishna in a wrestling match. In the arena, it was Krishna who triumphed, killing Chanur. *from: Shrimad Bhagavatam.*

chapati: unleavened Indian bread.

chidakash: the subtle space of Consciousness in the *sahasrara* and in the heart.

chin mudra: hand gesture in which the tip of the thumb and index finger touch while the other three fingers are outstretched, practiced during meditation to keep spiritual energy from flowing out of the body.

Chiti (*or*: Chitshakti, Kundalini, Kundalini Shakti, Mahamaya, Parashakti, Shakti): divine conscious energy; creative aspect of God, portrayed as the universal Mother.

Chitshakti: the power of universal Consciousness. *see also*: Chiti.

darshan: seeing or being in the presence of a revered person, sacred idol or sacred place.

Dasharatha: King of Ayodhya and father of Rama.

Dattatreya: a divine incarnation known as the Lord of *avadhutas,* and often revered as the embodiment of the supreme Guru.

Daulatabad Fort: a fort in the Deccan plateau in central Maharashtra which was built by the Hindu kings in the twelfth century. It was at this fort that the poet-saint Eknath Maharaj served his discipleship under his Guru Janardan Swami.

dharma: essential duty; religion; the law of righteousness.

dhoti: common dress for men in India, a length of material wrapped around the waist.

Dhruva: boy who performed severe penance to gain a high and eternal position. He became the polestar by the grace of Vishnu.

dhup: fragrant incense made from herbs, plants, and flowers burned as an offering in worship.

dhyana: meditation. *see also*: eight limbs of yoga.

Diksha: any religious initiation; initiation given by a Guru usually by imparting a mantra; in Siddha Yoga it means the spiritual awakening of the disciple by Shaktipat. *see also*: Siddha Yoga, Shaktipat.

Durga (*lit.* hard to conquer): one of the names of the universal Mother. In Her personal form, She is portrayed as an eight-armed goddess who rides a lion and carries weapons. She is the destroyer of evil tendencies.

Dwarka: one of the major pilgrimage centers of India, the ancient capitol of Krishna's kingdom.

eight limbs of yoga (*or*: Ashtanga Yoga, Raja Yoga): the eight-fold yoga expounded by Patanjali in his *Yoga Sutras*, the authoritative text on Raja Yoga. The eight steps are:

1. *yamas*: the practice of five moral virtues—non-violence, truthfulness, celibacy, nonstealing, and noncovetousness.

2. *niyamas*: the practice of five regular habits—purity, contentment, austerity, study, and surrender.

3. *asana*: posture.

4. *pranayama*: the regulation and restraint of breath.

5. *pratyahara*: withdrawal of the mind from sense objects.

6. *dharana*: concentration, fixing the mind on an object of contemplation.

7. *dhyana*: meditation, the continuous flow of thoughts toward one object.

8. *samadhi*: complete absorption or identification with the object of meditation, meditative union with the Absolute.

Eknath Maharaj (1528-1609): householder poet-saint of Maharashtra, the illustrious disciple of Janardan Swami, who in his later life became renowned for his scriptural commentaries and his spiritual poetry.

five elements:　ether, air, fire, water, earth; these comprise the elemental basis of the universe.

five sheaths:　the five coverings of an embodied soul, which determine the personality and nature of individual consciousness. They are: *annamaya kosha*—the food sheath, composed of gross matter which constitutes the gross body; *pranamaya kosha*—the five vital airs and five organs of action, i.e. organs of speech, grasping, locomotion, excretion, and generation; *manomaya kosha*—the mind and the five senses of perception; *vijnanamaya kosha*—the intellect; and *anandamaya kosha*—the bliss sheath, composed of ignorance.

Ganapati (*or*: Ganesha):　the elephant-headed god, son of Shiva and Parvati, who is the destroyer of sorrows and the remover of obstacles.

Ghirishneshwar:　a temple sacred to Shiva, built in the eighteenth century by Queen Ahalyabai, located in central Maharashtra.

Girnar Mountain:　a sacred mountain situated in Gujarat, considered to be the abode of many great Siddhas, including Lord Dattatreya and Gorakhnath.

Gita (*or: Bhagavad Gita*):　one of the essential scriptures of Hinduism, a portion of the *Mahabharata,* in which Krishna instructs Arjuna on the battlefield on the nature of God, universe and Self, on the different forms of yoga, and on the way to attain God. *see also: Mahabharata.*

Gokul:　a town in North India where Krishna spent his boyhood as the son of Nanda, a cowherd.

gopis:　the milkmaids of Vraja, childhood companions and devotees of Krishna. They are revered as the embodiments of the ideal states of ecstatic devotion to God.

Gorakhnath:　one of the nine Naths, a lineage of yogis known for their extraordinary powers. Gorakhnath was the Guru of Gahininath, who initiated Nivrittinath, Jnaneshwar's older brother and Guru.

gunas:　the three basic qualities of nature, which determine the inherent characteristics of all created things. They are: *sattva*—purity, light, harmony; *rajas*—activity, passion; and *tamas*—dullness, inertia, ignorance.

gurubhava: absorption in the Guru, identification with the Guru.

Gurudev: a term of address for the Guru, signifying the Guru as an embodiment of God.

Guru Gita (lit. song of the Guru): a garland of mantras in the form of a dialogue between Shiva and His consort Parvati, which explains the identity of the Guru with the supreme Absolute and describes the nature of the Guru, the Guru/disciple relationship, and meditation on the Guru.

gurukripa (lit. Guru's grace): the divine energy bestowed on a seeker through the compassion of the Guru.

Guru Om: the mantra by which the inner Self is remembered in the form of the Guru.

hamsa gayatri mantra: a sacred mantra from the *Vedas.*

Hanuman: the ideal bhakta and servant of Rama, in the form of a monkey of great strength. *from: Ramayana.*

Hara: a name for Shiva.

Hari (*also*: Lord Hari): a name for Vishnu.

Hatha Yoga: a yogic discipline by which the *samadhi* state is attained by uniting the *prana* and *apana* (ingoing and outgoing breath). Various bodily and mental exercises are practiced for the purpose of purifying the 72,000 *nadis* and to bring about the even flow of *prana.* When the flow of *prana* is even, the mind becomes still. One then experiences equality-consciousness and enters into the state of *samadhi.*

Hatha Yoga Pradipika: authoritative treatise on Hatha Yoga, written by Svatmarama Yogi, in which the practice of various Hatha Yoga techniques, such as *pranayama, asanas, mudras,* etc. are described.

Himalayas: the tallest range of mountains in the world, located along the boarder of India and China, which are considered to be the sacred abode of yogis, sages and gods.

householders: *see: ashramas.*

initiation: *see: diksha.*

Janaka: saintly king of Mithila in ancient India, the father of Sita, Lord Rama's consort.

Janardan Swami (1504-1575): a saint of Maharashtra who was appointed by the Mohammedan king as commander-in-chief of the Daulatabad fort. He devoted himself to the service of God while performing wordly duties. He was the Guru of the famous Maharashtrian poet-saint, Eknath Maharaj.

japa: repetition of a mantra.

jivanmukti: one who is liberated while still in the physical body.

jivatma: individual soul.

Jnaneshwar Maharaj (1275-1296): foremost among the saints of Maharashtra and a child yogi of extraordinary powers. Born in a family of saints, his older brother Nivrittinath, was his guru. His verse commentary on the *Gita*, the *Jnaneshwari*, written in the Marathi language is acknowledged as one of the world's most important spiritual works. He also composed a short work, *Amritanubhava,* and over 100 *abhangas* in which he describes various spiritual experiences of the Siddha Path. He took live *samadhi* at the age of 21 in Alandi, where his *samadhi* shrine continues to attract thousands of seekers to this day.

Jnaneshwari (or: Bhavartha Dipika): Jnaneshwar Maharaj's commentary on the *Bhagavad Gita* written in Marathi verse when he was 16 years old.

jnani: an enlightened being; a follower of the path of knowledge (*jnana*).

Kabir (1440-1518): a great poet-saint who lived his life as a weaver in Benares. His ecstatic poems describe the experience of the Self, the greatness of the Guru, and the nature of true spirituality. His followers were both Hindus and Moslems, and his influence was a strong force in overcoming religious factionalism.

Kakabhushandi: a sage of ancient times who was cursed by Shiva to become a crow. Through his constant devotion to Rama, he attained liberation. *from: Ramacaritamanasa* by Tulsidas.

Kailasa: a mountain peak in the Himalayas (in present-day Tibet) revered as the abode of Shiva.

kala: a small part, a digit, 1/16 of the whole.

Kamsa: wicked ruler of Mathura who was killed by his nephew, Krishna. *from: Shrimad Bhagavatam.*

Kannada: the main language of Karnataka state in South India.

karma: physical, verbal, or mental action. *see also: prarabdha karma.*

Kashi (*or*: Varanasi, Benares): a holy city sacred to Shiva located in North India on the banks of the Ganges River. According to Hindu tradition, whoever dies in this city attains liberation.

Kashmir Shaivism: nondual philosophy that recognizes the entire universe as a manifestation of Chiti, or divine conscious energy. Kashmir Shaivism explains how the formless, unmanifest supreme principle, manifests as the universe. The authoritative scripture of Kashmir Shaivism is the *Shiva Sutras,* a Sanskrit text consisting of seventy-seven sutras, attributed to Shiva and revealed to the sage, Vasuguptacharya.

Kasyapa: grandson of Brahma, the creator.

Kaushalya: mother of Rama and queen of Dasharatha.

khichari: Indian dish prepared from rice and lentils.

kinnaras: celestial musicians.

knot of the heart: *see*: three knots.

Krishna (*lit.* the dark one; the one who attracts irresistibly): the eighth incarnation of Vishnu, whose life story is described in the *Shrimad Bhagavatam* and the *Mahabharata,* and whose spiritual teachings are contained in the *Bhagavad Gita.*

kriyas: gross (physical) or subtle (mental, emotional) purificatory movements initiated by the awakened Kundalini. *Kriyas* purify the body and nervous system so as to allow a seeker to endure the energy of higher states of consciousness.

kumbhaka: voluntary or involuntary retention of breath.

kumkum: red-colored powder, made from tumeric, used for putting the auspicious mark between the eyebrows in remembrance of the Guru, and for ritual worship.

Kundalini (*lit.* coiled one): the primordial Shakti or cosmic energy that lies coiled in the *muladhara chakra* of every individual. When awakened, Kundalini begins to move upward within the *sushumna,* the subtle central channel, piercing the *chakras* and initiating various yogic processes which bring about total purification and rejuvenation of the entire being. When Kundalini enters the *sahasrara,* the spiritual center in the crown of the head, the individual self merges in the universal Self and attains the state of Self-realization.

kutir: hut.

Lakshmi: the goddess of wealth and prosperity and the consort of Vishnu.

liberation: freedom from the cycle of birth and death; state of realization of oneness with the supreme Consciousness.

loka (*lit.* world): plane of existence, both physical and subtle.

lungi: common dress for men in India, a piece of cloth tied around the waist.

Mahabharata: the epic poem compiled by the sage Vyasa which recounts the struggle between the Kaurava and the Pandava brothers over a disputed kingdom. As its vast narrative unfolds, a treasure-house of Indian secular and religious lore is revealed. The *Bhagavad Gita* occurs in the latter portion of the *Mahabharata.*

Mahadeva (*lit.* great god): a name of Shiva.

Mahamaya (*lit.* the great illusion): a name of Shakti. *see also*: Chiti, Shakti.

Mahesha (*lit.* great lord): a name of Shiva.

Mandaleshwar: title conferred upon well-known and respected *sannyasi* who heads an ashram or monastery, and who is the chief of *sannyasis* of a particular region.

mandir: temple.

mantra: sacred words or mystical cosmic sounds; God in the form of sound.

Manu: the lawgiver of Indian tradition.

maya: the force that shows the unreal as real, and presents what is temporary and short-lived as eternal and everlasting. The force that conceals our divinity.

Mira (1433-1468): a Rajasthani queen and poet-saint famous for her poems of devotion to Krishna. She was so absorbed in her love for Krishna that when she was fed poison by diaspproving relatives, the poison turned to nectar.

mridang: a two-headed South Indian drum, which provides the rhythm for *kirtan,* group chanting of God's name.

mudra: various advanced Hatha Yoga techniques practiced to hold the *prana* within the body, forcing the Kundalini to flow into the *sushumna.* These *mudras* can occur spontaneously after receiving Shaktipat; symbolic gestures and movements of the hands, which express inner feelings and inner states, or which convey various meanings such as: charity, knowledge, and fearlessness. Many deities, saints, and idols are pictured performing these gestures granting their benediction.

muladhara chakra: the *chakra* at the base of the spine where Kundalini lies coiled like a snake. From Her seat at *muladhara*, Kundalini controls all the activities of the physiological system through its network of 72,000 nerves. *see also: chakra.*

nada: divine music or sound which is heard in higher states of meditation.

nadis: the 72,000 channels of vital force in the body.

Namdev (1270-1350): poet-saint of Pandharpur in Maharashtra, a tailor by caste and contemporary of Jnaneshwar Maharaj. He was a devotee of Lord Vitthal and had realized God in His personal form, but he could not realize the all-pervasive nature of God until he met his Guru, Visoba Khechar. He composed thousands of devotional songs, many of which glorify the repetition of the divine name.

Nanak (*also*: Guru Nanak, Nanakdev; 1469-1538):   The first Guru and founder of the Sikh religion. He traveled widely, teaching liberal religious and social doctrines.

Narada: a divine *rishi,* or seer, a great devotee and servant of Vishnu. He appears in many of the *Puranas* and is the author of the *Narada Bhakti Sutras*, the authoritative text on Bhakti Yoga.

nataraja (*lit.* king of dance):   an epithet of Shiva, referred to as the dancing Shiva. The object of His dance is to free all souls from the fetters of illusion. The whole cosmic play, or *lila*, is the dance of Shiva. All movements within the cosmos are His dance. He sets into motion the creation of the world, and when the time comes, also destroys all names and forms through His dancing.

nine jewels: nine precious jewels, including pearl and coral, which are frequently mentioned in the scriptures.

nine openings: the nine openings in the body: eyes, ears, nose, mouth, anus, and sexual organ.

nirguna: without attribute, the formless aspect of God.

nirvikalpa: the highest state of *samadhi,* beyond all thought, attribute, and description.

Om: the primal sound; sound or vibration from which the entire universe emanates. It is the inner essence of all mantras.

Om Namah Shivaya: a mantra, meaning "Salutations to Shiva." Shiva denotes the inner Self. The mantra *Namah Shivaya* consists of five letters and is called *panchakshari* mantra. It is known as the great redeeming mantra because it has the power to grant worldly fulfillment as well as spiritual realization.

padmasana (*lit.* lotus posture):   the most important posture for meditation, formed by sitting on the ground with the back erect, placing the right foot over the left thigh and the left foot over the right thigh. Both hands can be placed on the knee joints.

Paramatma (*lit.* supreme Self):   a name of God.

Parameshvara (*lit.* supreme Lord):   a name of God.

Parashakti (*lit.* supreme Shakti):   the Absolute in its form as dynamic, creative energy.

Parashara: grandson of Vasishtha, who while crossing the river Yamuna in the boat of a fisherwoman was overwhelmed by passion
for her. The sage Vyasa was born as a result of their union.

Parashiva (*lit.* supreme Shiva):   the primal Lord; the supreme Guru.

Parvati (*lit.* daughter of the mountains):   wife of Shiva and daughter
of the King of the Himalayas; a name of the universal Mother or
Shakti.

philosopher's stone: a jewel which is said to have the power to trans-
mute base metals into gold.

prakriti: nature; material cause of creation according to Sankhya
philosophy. *see also*: six schools of Indian philosophy.

pranava: the word which refers to the mystic syllable *Om. see also:
Om.*

pranayama: the regulation and restraint of breath. *see also*: eight
limbs of yoga.

prarabdha karma: accumulated past actions, the fruits of which are
experienced now and cannot be erased.

prasad: a gift from God; an offering made to God which is then distributed to devotees with His blessings.

Pratyabhijnahridayam (*lit.* the heart of the doctrine of recognition):
a concise treatise of twenty sutras by Kshemaraja which sum-
marizes the Pratyabhijna philosophy of Kashmir Shaivism. In
essence it states that man has forgotten his true nature by identifying with the body. Realization is a process of recognizing our
true nature.   Swami Muktananda has commented on these sutras
in the book, *Siddha Meditation. see also*: Kashmir Shaivism.

Puranas (*lit.* ancient legends):   there are 18 *Puranas,* or sacred books,
containing stories, legends, and hymns about the creation of the
universe, the incarnations of God, and the instructions of various
deities as well as the spiritual legacies of ancient sages and kings.

puris: deep-fried Indian bread.

purusha (*lit.* person):   the individual soul; the indwelling form of God.

Putana: demoness who was sent by Kamsa to kill the baby Krishna
by suckling him on her breasts, which were smeared with poison.
While sucking her milk, Krishna sucked out her breath and killed
her. As a result, she attained liberation.

Radha: the childhood companion and consort of Krishna who is
celebrated in Indian tradition as the embodiment of devotion to
God.

Raja Yoga: *see*: eight limbs of yoga.

rajas: *see: gunas.*

Rama: the seventh incarnation of Vishnu, whose life story is told in the *Ramayana* epic; a name of the all-pervasive Supreme Reality. *see also: Ramayana.*

Ramayana (*lit.* history of Rama): the oldest of the Sanskrit epic poems written by the sage Valmiki. The *Ramayana* celebrates the life and exploits of Rama, the seventh incarnation of Vishnu. The story tells of the abduction of Sita, Rama's wife, by the ten-headed demon king Ravana, and how Rama, along with the help of Hanuman and the monkey kingdom, fought and conquered Ravana.

Rameshwaram: a sacred place in South India, where Rama worshipped a *shivalingam* in preparation for his battle with the demon king Ravana. It is one of the major places of pilgrimage in India today. *see also: shivalingam.*

Rudra: a name of Shiva.

Rudrahridaya Upanishad: one of the *Shaiva Upanishads,* which identifies Shiva with the Absolute. *see also: Upanishads.*

rudraksha: seeds from a tree sacred to Shiva strung as beads for rosaries.

sacred thread: thread worn over one shoulder indicating the religious initiation of the *brahmin, kshatriya,* and *vaishya* castes. *see also*: caste.

Sadguru: the true Guru; a perfect Master.

sadhaka: an aspirant on the spiritual path.

sadhana: the practice of spiritual discipline.

sadhu: a monk or ascetic.

sahaja: natural; that which occurs naturally or spontaneously.

sahasrara: the topmost spiritual center or thousand-petaled lotus located in the crown of the head. It is the seat of Shiva, the supreme Guru. When Kundalini Shakti unites with Shiva in the *sahasrara,* the yogi achieves the state of Self-realization.

Sai Baba of Shirdi (1838-1918): one of the great Siddhas of modern times. His *samadhi* shrine, at Shirdi, is a popular place of pilgrimage.

samadhi: a state of meditative union with the Absolute. *see also*: eight limbs of yoga.

samadhi shrine: site where a saint has taken *mahasamadhi;* the tomb of a saint, which is alive with the spiritual power of the saint who is buried there.

samsara: the cycle of birth and death; worldly illusion.

Sanjaya: the narrator of the *Bhagavad Gita.*

sannyasa: *see: ashramas.*

sannyasi: an ascetic ordained as a monk, a renunciant, who has taken the formal vows of renunciation.

satchidananda: the nature of the supreme reality. *sat* is Being, that which exists in all times, in all places, and in all things; *chit* is Consciousness, that which illumines all things; and *ananda* is supreme Bliss.

satsang: a meeting of devotees to hear scriptures, chant, or sit in the presence of a holy being; the company of saints and devotees.

sattva: *see: gunas.*

seed letter (seed mantra):   a basic sound from the Sanskrit language the repetition of which manifests the object, deity, or state which it represents.

seven bodily components: lymphatic fluid, flesh, bone, blood marrow, semen, and fat.

seven sages: Atri, Gautama, Vasishtha, Bharadwaja, Kashyapa, Vishvamitra, and Jamadagni; there are seven sages who are born in each world cycle.

Shaivism: the worship of Shiva as the supreme Self; the philosophical school which describes the nature of reality as the all-pervasive Shiva. *see also*: Kashmir Shaivism.

Shaivite: one who worships Shiva as the supreme Self.

Shakti (*or*: Chiti, Kundalini, Kundalini Shakti):   force; energy; the divine cosmic energy which projects, maintains, and dissolves the universe; spouse of Shiva. *see also*: Chiti, Kundalini.

Shaktipat: transmission of spiritual power (Shakti) from the Guru to disciple; spiritual awakening by grace.

shambhavi mudra: a state of spontaneous *samadhi* in which the eyes become focused within although they remain half-open; the state of supreme Shiva.

Shandilya: ancient seer who wrote *Shandilya Bhakti Sutras*, a treatise on *bhakti.*

Shankaracharya (788-820):   the great Indian philosopher and saint, who expounded the philosophy of absolute nondualism (Advaita Vedanta). He traveled all over India defeating the contending schools of philosophy and revived Hinduism and established *maths* (ashrams) in the four corners of India.

Shaunaka: ancient sage who commented on the *Vedas.*

Shesha: the divine serpent who upholds the earth on his mantle.

Shiva: a name for the all-pervasive supreme Reality; one of the Hindu trinity of gods, representing God as the destroyer; the personal God of the Shaivites. In his personal form, he is portrayed as a yogi wearing a tiger skin and holding a trident, with snakes coiled around his neck and arms.

Shiva's armor: a group of mantras sacred to Shiva, which secure His protection.

Shiva's army: a host of strange beings, ghosts, phantoms, and demoniacal creatures who attend Shiva.

Shiva Drishti (*lit.* the outlook of Shiva):   a text of Kashmir Shaivism by Somananda written in the tenth century. *see also*: Kashmir Shaivism.

shivalingam: phallic-shaped symbol of Shiva representing the impersonal aspect of God.

Shiva Samhita: a Sanskrit text on yoga which describes the correspondence of the macrocosm (universe) and the microcosm (human body) as well as an explanation of the practice of *asanas, pranayama,* and *mudras,* in order to awaken the Kundalini.

Shiva Sutras: a Sanskrit text which Shiva revealed to the sage Vasuguptacharya. It consists of seventy-seven sutras which were found inscribed on a rock in Kashmir. It is the scriptural authority for the philosophical school of Kashmir Shaivism. *see also*: Kashmir Shaivism.

Shivo'ham: a mantra, meaning "I am Shiva."

Shree Gurudev Ashram: former name of Gurudev Siddha Peeth, the Ashram of Swami Muktananda Paramahamsa in Ganeshpuri, outside of Bombay.

Shrimad Bhagavatam: the most popular devotional scripture in India containing many legends, stories, and the life and teachings of Krishna. It was composed by Vyasa.

Shuka (Shukadeva):   a great sage of ancient times, the son of Vyasa. He is mentioned in many scriptures, but is most famous as the narrator of the *Shrimad Bhagavatam. see also: Shrimad Bhagavatam.*

Shyama (*lit.* the dark one):   a name of Krishna, so-called because of his dark blue complexion.

Siddha: perfect human being; one who has attained the state of unity awareness; who experiences himself as all-pervasive and who has achieved mastery over his senses and their objects.

Siddharudha Swami: saint in whose ashram Swami Muktananda stayed for some time in Hubli, Mysore State.

siddhasana (*lit.* the perfect posture): a posture used for meditation formed by placing one heel at the anus and placing the other heel at the root of the sexual organ, with the ankle joints touching one another.

siddhis: supernatural powers attained through mantra repetition, meditation, and other yogic practices. The eight major *siddhis* are:

1. *anima*: ability to reduce one's body to the size of an atom—this *siddhi* is used to travel to subtle realms.

2. *mahima*: ability to expand the body to any size.

3. *laghima*: ability to make the body light—levitation.

4. *garima*: ability to make the body heavy.

5. *prapti*: ability to attain everything.

6. *prakamya*: ability to see one's wishes fulfilled.

7. *ishatva*: ability to gain lordship over everything.

8. *vashitva*: power to attract and control all things.

Sita: a name of the universal Mother; wife of Rama and a symbol of wifely devotion.

six schools of Indian philosophy: the six philosophical schools of thought which base their teachings on the authority of the *Vedas*. They are:

1. Nyaya, founded by Gautama, is the school of logical proof.

2. Vaishesika, written down by Kanada, teaches knowledge of reality is attained by understanding nine basic essences which comprise existence.

3. Sankhya, founded by Kapilamuni, attempts to harmonize the philosophy of the *Vedas* through reason and views the world as comprised of two ultimate realities: Spirit (*purusha*) and Matter (*prakriti*).

4. Yoga, expounded by Patanjali in his *Yoga Sutras*, shows the practical means to attain union with God by following an eight-limbed path. *see also*: eight limbs of yoga.

5. Purva Mimamsa, written down by Jaimini, interprets how the actions enjoined by the *Vedas* lead to liberation.

6. Uttara Mimamsa or Vedanta, founded by Badarayana, contains the philosophical teachings of the *Upanishads*, which investigate the nature and relationship of Brahman, the world, and the Self.

So'ham (*lit.* I am That): the natural vibration of the Self, which occurs spontaneously with each incoming and outgoing breath.

By becoming aware of it, a yogi experiences the identity between his individual self and the supreme Self.

Spanda Shastras: a body of philosophical works in Kashmir Shaivism which elaborate the principles of the *Shiva Sutras* using logical reason in support of them. *see also*: Kashmir Shaivism, *Shiva Sutras.*

sri: a term of respect; also means wealth, prosperity, glory, success— the term means master of all these.

Sri Sailam: a holy place near Hyderabad in South India, known as an abode of Siddhas.

Sudama: a childhood friend and devotee of Krishna.

Sundardas (1596-1689): a renowned Hindu poet-saint, born in Rajasthan.

Surdas (1479-1584): Blind poet-saint. Devoted to child Krishna, he spent his life in Vraja. The legend has it that once when his eyes followed a beautiful woman, he took a tamboura string and put them out.

sushumna: the central and most important of all 72,000 *nadis* located in the center of the spinal column extending from the base of the spine to the top of the head. The six *chakras* are situated in the *sushumna* and it is through the *sushumna* channel that the Kundalini rises. *see also: chakra,* Kundalini, *nadi.*

Suta: hermit and disciple of Vyasa who narrated the *Puranas* to other hermits.

Sutapa: one of the *prajapatis,* or divine beings, who assisted Brahma in the creation of the world.

tamas: *see: gunas.*

tamboura: a four-stringed musical instrument which plays the drone accompaniment in Indian music.

tantra: an esoteric spiritual discipline which worships Shakti, the creative power of the Absolute, as the divine Mother through the practice of rituals, mantras, and *yantras.* The goal of *tantra* is attaining Self-realization through Kundalini awakening and through uniting the two principles, Shiva and Shakti.

Tantras: divinely revealed scriptures in the form of dialogues between Shiva and Parvati, revealing the secrets of knowledge, meditation, and devotion to the Guru, and practices for the attainment of Self-realization.

tapasya (or: tapa; lit. to heat up): austere or ascetic practices, which purify the mind and give control over the senses.

thirty-six principles (*tattvas*):   according to Kashmir Shaivism, the thirty-six stages in which the unmanifest supreme principle manifests in the universe. *see also*: Kashmir Shaivism.

three knots (*granthis*):   the three junction points in the *sushumna* where the *ida, pingala,* and *sushumna nadis* converge and form a knot. They are: *Brahma granthi*—located in the *muladhara chakra; Vishnu granthi*—located in the *anahata* (heart) *chakra;* and *Rudra granthi*—located in the *ajna chakra.* When Kundalini is awakened, She pierces through these knots as She ascends upward to the *sahasrara.*

three worlds: the three worlds referred to in the scriptures are: heaven, earth, and hell.

tonga: two-wheeled horse-drawn carriage.

Tukaram Maharaj (1608-1650):   great poet-saint of Maharashtra born at Dehu. He received initiation in a dream from a saint from Siddhaloka. He wrote thousands of *abhangas* (devotional songs) many of which describe his *sadhana* and spiritual experiences, his initiation, his realization, and the glory of the divine name.

tulsi: a plant sacred to Vishnu, a type of basil whose leaves are used for worship.

Tulsidas (1532-1623):   North Indian poet-saint and author of *Ramacaritamanasa,* the life story of Rama written in Hindi, which is still one of the most popular scriptures in India today.

turiya: the transcendental state, the fourth state of consciousness beyond waking, dream, and deep sleep, in which the true nature of reality is directly perceived; the state of Witness-consciousness.

turiyatita: the state beyond *turiya*; the supremely blissful state of complete freedom from all duality and the awareness of the one Self in all, the final attainment of Siddha Yoga.

Uddhava: friend and devotee of Krishna. Krishna imparted His teachings to Uddhava in Book Eleven of the *Shrimad Bhagavatam,* referred to as *Uddhava Gita.*

Uma: a name for Shakti, the consort of Shiva, meaning light. This aspect represents the power to illuminate or pure knowledge.

Upanishads: the teachings of the ancient sages which form the knowledge or the end portion of the *Vedas.* The central teaching of the *Upanishads* is that the Self of man is the same as Brahman, the Absolute. The goal of life, according to the *Upanishads,* is realization of Brahman.

Vaikuntha: the celestial abode of Vishnu.

Vaishnava: related to Vishnu.

Vaishnavite: one who worships Vishnu as the supreme Self.

Varuna: the god of waters and the guardian of the western quarter of the universe.

Vasuguptacharya (ninth century):   the sage to whom Shiva revealed the *Shiva Sutras. see also*: Kashmir Shaivism, *Shiva Sutras.*

Vedanta (*lit.* the end of the *Veda*):   *see*: six schools of Indian philosophy.

Vedas: the four ancient, authoritative Hindu scriptures, regarded as divinely revealed. They contain: hymns in praise of gods, sacrificial prayers, codes of conduct for religious and social life, treatises relating to prayer and sacrificial ceremonies, and the mystic teachings of ancient sages. The four *Vedas* are: *Rig Veda, Yajur Veda, Sama Veda,* and *Athara Veda.*

veena: a stringed instrument.

Vibhishana: brother of the demon king, Ravana, and a devotee of Lord Rama.

Vidura: a devotee of Krishna.

vidya: learning, knowledge, science.

Vishnu: a name for the all-pervasive supreme Reality; one of the Hindu trinity of gods, representing God as the sustainer; the personal God of the Vaishnavas. In His personal form, He is portrayed as four-armed holding a conch, a discus, a lotus, and a mace. He is dark blue in color. During times of great wickedness and trouble, Vishnu incarnates on the earth in order to protect men and gods and reestablish righteousness. There are ten such incarnations in our present world cycle, Rama and Krishna being the most important.

vishuddha chakra: *see: chakra.*

Vitthal (*lit.* the place of the brick):   Krishna went to the house of Pundalik, who while tending to his aged parents asked Him to wait and threw a brick for Him to stand on. This form of Krishna standing on a brick is known as Vitthal. His image is enshrined in Pandharpur, a famous place of pilgrimage in Maharashtra, and was worshiped by the poet-saints of Maharashtra and Karnataka.

Vraja: a district on the banks of the Yamuna River where Krishna lived and sported with the *gopis.*

Vyasa: a great sage of ancient times, compiler of the *Vedas, Puranas,* and author of the *Mahabharata.* He is the father of Shukamuni.

Wish-fulfilling cow: the sacred cow, considered to be a goddess who has the power to give milk whenever needed by gods and sages, and who grants one's wishes.

Wish-fulfilling jewel: a diamond, salvaged from the ocean of milk, which has the power to grant one's wishes. *from: Shrimad Bhagavatam.*

Wish-fulfilling tree: a heavenly tree that has the power to grant the wish of anyone standing under it.

Yajnavalkya: a sage whose teachings are recorded in the *Brihadaranyaka Upanishad,* the Guru of King Janaka.

yakshas: a class of semi-divine beings whose king, Kubera, is the lord of wealth.

Yamaraj: the god of death.

Yamuna River: a holy river which flows in North India on the banks of which Krishna spent his youth and sported with the *gopis*. The place where the Yamuna meets the Ganges River is revered as a sacred spot and is a pilgrimage center. *see also*: Allahabad.

yoga (*lit*. union):   the state of oneness with the Self, God; the practices leading to that state.

yogi: one who practices yoga; one who has attained the goal of yogic practices.

Yogashikha Upanishad: one of the *Yoga Upanishads* which discusses the path of knowledge in all its aspects and expounds the subject of yoga as an aid to knowledge. *see also: Upanishads.*

yogini: a female practitioner of yoga.

Index

OTHER PUBLICATIONS

BY GURUMAYI CHIDVILASANANDA
Ashes At My Guru's Feet
Kindle My Heart, Volumes I & II

BY SWAMI MUKTANANDA
From the Finite to the Infinite, Volumes I & II
I Am That
Kundalini: The Secret of Life
Secret of the Siddhas
Siddha Meditation
I Have Become Alive
Does Death Really Exist?
Getting Rid of What You Haven't Got
Where Are You Going?
Light on the Path
The Perfect Relationship
Mukteshwari I & II
Satsang With Baba, Volumes I-V
Reflections of the Self
In the Company of a Siddha
Mystery of the Mind
Meditate
I Love You
To Know the Knower
The Self Is Already Attained
A Book for the Mind
I Welcome You All With Love
God Is With You

Siddha Meditation is practiced in more than 600 Ashrams and Centers around the world. For information, contact:
Gurudev Siddha Peeth
P.O. Ganeshpuri (PIN 401206)
District Thana, Maharashtra, India
or Centers Office, SYDA Foundation
P.O. Box 600, South Fallsburg, NY 12779
(914) 434-2000